Letters to Doctors:

Patients Educating Medical Professionals Through Practical True-Life Experiences

The BRCA and Hereditary Breast and Ovarian Cancer Syndrome Edition

Dr. Jonathan D. Herman

Teri Smieja

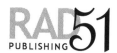

Letters to Doctors:
Patients Educating Medical Professionals through Practical True-Life Experiences

Dr. Jonathan D. Herman & Teri Smieja
ISBN-13: 978-1-939776-29-7
ISBN-10: 1939776295

10 9 8 7 6 5 4 3 2 1
First Edition

Published in the United States.

Cover Model: Teri Smieja
Photography of Ms. Smieja: Koryn Hutchinson Photography

Cover Art Design: Farah Evers Designs
www.FarahEvers.com

Interior Book Design: Accentuate Services
Editing: Derek Odom & Michelle Devon
Proofing: Teri Smieja, Derek Odom & Lynn Hunter

Acknowledgements

Many thanks to the members of the BRCA Sisterhood and commenters of the blog, *Teri's Blip in the Universe*, who, without their input, this book could not have been written.

Teri

A special thanks to my family for putting up with, accepting, and loving me more for my BRCA advocacy.

Dr. Herman

Special thanks to Dr. Herman's patients, colleagues, friends and family for their input, advice and personal stories.

Disclaimer

Letters to Doctors is provided for informational purposes only and should not be relied upon for diagnosis and/or treatment. The contents are not intended to replace professional medical advice. Always utilize evidence-based medical information for questions regarding any medical condition. Never base medical diagnosis or delay treatment because of information in *Letters to Doctors*.

Specific diagnostic or therapeutic procedures and/or treatment modalities, including but not limited to: surgery, medication, or products mentioned in this book, are neither endorsed nor recommended by *Letters to Doctors*, its contributors or authors. *Letters to Doctors* does not assume liability for the contents or material provided in this book.

Reliance on information provided by *Letters to Doctors* is solely at your own risk. *Letters to Doctors* accepts no liability or responsibility for damages or injuries arising from use of any product, information, idea, or instruction contained in the materials mentioned herein.

Please be advised: *Because of the nature of this book and the issues Letters to Doctors addresses, this book contains material that is anatomically and sexually explicit, and therefore, might be offensive to some people.*

More than the Sum

I am more than the sum of my body parts,
I consist of light, grace, and soul.
The lilt of my laugh, the touch of my hand,
The sound of my voice, and the timber of my heart.
I am not the shape of my leg,
But instead the path of my walk,
I am not the size of my breasts,
But I am the consistency of the heart the lies beneath them.
My womb is not measured by the children I birth,
But by the birth I give to the life around me,
I am not the scars and lines that mar my face and body,
But they are the medals of life and honor I wear with pride.
I am not the color and style of my hair or skin,
But the intelligence and creativity that works beneath it,
I am not the slightness or weight that fits in my clothes,
But the size of the humanity who makes a mark in my world.
No part removed makes me any less of a perfectly formed person,
For no individual piece can hold all that I am,
I am mother, sister, teacher, lover, grandchild, friend, daughter and wife,

I am all of these and more, a work of creation and beauty.
Woman.

~~ LL Darroch

Table of Contents

Preface

This original book combines the perspective of a practicing Obstetrics/Gynecologist and a BRCA1 positive patient who met online. Through their mutual desire to help people who live with the threat or actuality of BRCA mutations and Hereditary Breast and Ovarian Cancer Syndrome (HBOC), Dr. Herman and Teri Smieja have become HBOC/BRCA advocates and work tirelessly to inform, educate, and empower those faced with hereditary cancers.

Merging the dynamics of a doctor and a patient who share a common goal of educating not just patients, but healthcare professionals, too, results in an easy to read, hard to put down book that's been written specifically for the healthcare professional, making this a book like no other in the HBOC/BRCA realm.

It is their belief that physicians, nurse practitioners, physician assistants, and most of those working within the healthcare industry welcome education and constructive criticism, as long as it truly is well intended and presented in a positive and engaging manner.

By sharing their viewpoints, along with those of many women (and men) affected by HBOC and BRCA mutations, their goal is to give doctors and other medical professionals a valuable tool in helping to provide better and more specialized healthcare to the high cancer risk patient.

So many women have lost their breasts, their ovaries–their lives – to breast or ovarian cancer. Men with the BRCA mutation have battled breast cancer too. If only they had known of their BRCA mutation before they got sick.

~~**Teri Smieja**

It was my first time seeing the patient. I felt the breast mass and I just knew it was cancer. It didn't have to be. Her mother died from ovarian cancer and her grandmother had breast cancer. That history didn't happen yesterday.

~~**Jonathan Herman, MD**

That a woman may not have perfect breasts in no way detracts from her beauty. In fact, I'll be so bold as to say that it makes us even more lovely, as our scars unflinchingly show our strength, our ability to battle and win, and in the case of people such as myself, our beauty is made even more so, by our desire to put our lives above personal and societal vanity.

~~**Teri Smieja**

Introduction

Dr. Jonathan Herman

My journey into BRCA advocacy began on June 17, 2005. It has been over twenty years since I began my career as an OB/GYN. I no longer remember my first delivery, vaginal breech, or cesarean section; or my first crash C-section, abdominal hysterectomy or laparoscopic hysterectomy.

There are, however, a few select cases that remain as clear to me as the day they occurred. These cases are so remarkable, because they have had great impact in transforming the way I treat patients and practice medicine. One experience in particular stands out above all the rest.

In May 2005, I delivered a baby boy. The delivery was uncomplicated and in itself not out of the ordinary. Soon thereafter, the grandmother of that baby became my patient. She requested I remove her ovaries, because she tested positive for the breast cancer genetic mutation.

Back in 2005, I was aware of BRCA genetic mutations, but I hadn't knowingly been involved in the care of any of these patients.

On June 9, 2005, we went to the operating table. I performed a laparoscopic bilateral salpingo-oophorectomy (BSO) with washings. I burned the cornua with a Klepinger. I signed the pathology request form and made sure to highlight the words: **BRCA positive**.

Eight days later, on June 17, 2005 the report read, *"Ovary with poorly-differentiated carcinoma showing serous features. Prominent lymphovascular invasion present. Comment: The neoplastic ovary is almost completely replaced by carcinoma and measures .3cm in greatest diameter."*

At the time of surgery, the ovary had appeared normal.

This case shook me up a lot. If not for BRCA testing, this cancer would have gone undetected until metastatic. At that point, I became highly motivated. I attempted to learn all I could about hereditary breast and ovarian cancer syndrome (HBOC) and breast cancer (BRCA) testing. I read texts and journals. I searched for information on Medline and on websites like the National Institute of Health (NIH)[1] and American Society of Clinical Oncology (ASCO)[2].

By the beginning of 2006, I lectured in community forums and to healthcare providers. I encouraged them to identify patients who potentially carried a BRCA mutation. It became evident that one could only learn so much from the literature I was reading.

I thought I knew a lot at the time, but I began to understand so much more as I delved deeper into the subject. Every time I spoke, I learned something new. I acquired knowledge from colleagues who constantly challenged my understanding with worthwhile questions, and I learned even more from the patients themselves, who pointed to their concerns about real-world topics I had never even considered.

Over time, I gained new perspectives and greater insight into the BRCA world. BRCA-related blogs, websites, and Facebook groups are a great source of information. It is on the internet where I found ***Teri's Blip in the Universe***[3] and its blogger, my coauthor, Teri Smieja.

Early on, I thought I had learned about HBOC and BRCA. In retrospect, I see that, in 2005, I had just begun.

Teri Smieja, Patient Advocate
BRCA Previvor

I'm Teri Smieja (pronounced: Smaya), a forty-two-year-old married mother of two sons, one a college student and one in kindergarten.

Early in 2009, I tested positive for the BRCA1 genetic mutation (187delAG). I began blogging soon afterward for the main purpose of creating an outlet for my own feelings. It all came from an emotional level. In the beginning, when I first found out I had the mutation, I was confused, scared, totally lost, and I didn't know anything about BRCA genetic mutations at all.

Over time, that has changed.

I've learned so much and am no longer lost or alone. I continued to blog for a few years, for myself, but it became something more than just therapeutic writing for my own personal needs. I also used it in hopes of helping other women like myself, by sharing what I had learned and being open and honest about how I felt about what I was going through. It's amazing how similar most thoughts are regarding our mutations and pre-disposition to breast and ovarian cancer. We have so many of the same fears, worries, and questions. It is reassuring to know you aren't the only one to feel the way you feel.

It is a frightening thing to learn you have up to an eighty-seven-percent chance of getting breast cancer[4]. It's scary to be told you have up to a forty-four-percent chance of ovarian cancer (stats frequently given to a BRCA1-mutated person)[5]. Perhaps even scarier is to learn about the incredibly high recurrence rates of these cancers in the genetically mutated person. Metastatic cancers are, to me, the most frightening of all. Metastatic, of course, refers to cancer that originally started as another cancer. It could be looked at as the spin-off show of a sitcom. It was originally breast cancer (or ovarian, etc.) that was treated but comes back in the form of bone cancer, brain cancer, or any other type of cancer.

Along with my good friend, Karen Malkin-Lazarovitz, I co-created a support group on Facebook called the BRCA Sisterhood[6]. We had several close friends who also have a BRCA mutation who really helped to get this support group on the map. The group has been a wonderful success with nearly two thousand supportive members, all at varying ages and stages of their journey. In July of 2010 I was also honored enough to be asked by Facing our Risk of Cancer Empowered (FORCE)[7] to take the lead as the Social Network Coordinator on the Chase Community Giving Campaign[8]. Because of tireless efforts, FORCE was able to place in the top two hundred winning charities and won $20,000!

Taking charge of my life and putting myself in a position to help others has been a tremendously positive way for me and my family to handle my BRCA1 mutation.

The scientific crystal ball that is genetic testing has put me in the position to be able to take steps to potentially save myself from genetic breast and ovarian cancer. In October 2009, I had a bilateral salpingo-oophorectomy and a hysterectomy. A few months later, in February 2010, I had prophylactic bilateral mastectomy (PBM) with DIEP reconstruction. I went the skin sparing/nipple-sparing route. Unfortunately I ended up with complications: a delayed failure flap with the result of fat necrosis in my right breast.

In July 2010, I had a stage one hip flap do-over on my right side to reconstruct my right breast from scratch. A few weeks after the hip flap surgery, I developed a deep vein thrombosis (DVT, a blood clot) in my left calf. Part of it broke off and fragmented into many smaller clots that went into both sides of my lungs resulting in pulmonary emboli.

Not everyone has a cookie-cutter prophylactic surgery. In fact, few of us do! I finally finished my reconstruction in 2011 with an implant and fat injections in the right breast. I know my complications weren't in vain, as the very sharing of my experiences, both the positive and the negative, continues to be a great help to so many others.

About My Mom

April 27, 1953 – April 18, 1992

She was diagnosed with breast cancer at the young age of 35.
She left behind two daughters and a son at the young age of thirty-eight.
My mother rocked a bikini!
She made most of her own clothes.
She was a fashionista!
She threw really cool birthday parties!
Every birthday and Christmas she made me a new dress.
She even made me matching dresses for my Cabbage Patch dolls.
She had great breasts…then she only had one.
She had funny looking feet…because of all the stylish pointy high-heeled shoes she use to wear.
She could draw cool pictures.
She was attentive.
She loved to dance.
She always had great skin and a golden tan.
She had long legs and turned heads where ever she went.
She was careful.
Sometimes she didn't believe me.
She loved to camp.
She was self-conscious.
She was a great singer and sang in the church choir and cantatas.
She loved Jesus.
She used to clean houses.
She liked to go for walks.
She loved summer.
She was loved by everyone.
She had a great laugh.
She had great hair.
She was a real estate agent.
Sometimes, when she held my hand, she would walk too fast,
and I would have to run to keep up.
She read her bible.

She liked pork chops with applesauce.
She was my home.
She could be short tempered.
She adored her nieces and nephews.
She didn't like her teeth so she got braces.
She loved her teeth.
She went all out for Christmas and birthdays.
She could braid my hair so beautifully.
She felt alone.
She loved to plant marigolds and tomato plants.
She liked to eat cake batter and let us lick the bowl.
She made great Dutch soup.
She was a beach babe.
She had a vibrant smile.
She was a cat person.
She loved her children.
She cried during sad movies.
She suffered greatly.
She fought bravely.
She died tragically.
She died too young.

I wish I had more memories...

~~ Rachel H.
Author of "Losing the Boobs" Blog[9]

SECTION ONE

Who, What, When, Where and Why?

I'm No Longer Afraid

Dr. Jonathan Herman

I have spoken with thousands of practitioners about BRCA mutations while lecturing all over the United States. I have listened and responded to their concerns and questions. Teri, through her blog and Facebook group, the BRCA Sisterhood, has been vetting concerns of women from all over the world. The following chapters will highlight many of the topics we have encountered.

Using this valuable feedback, our objectives are as follows:

- *Provide information and viewpoints for practitioners*
- *Address and answer concerns posed by practitioners*
- *Address and answer questions patients have asked*
- *Relay constructive criticism*

I have asked many of my patients for their ideas, and Teri queried woman through her blog, the BRCA Sisterhood, and a special Facebook group she set up.

We hope you will take away a concept or two that will enhance your practice.

The first letter comes from Nikki M. (Texas). When she sent me her story, it made such an impact that we felt it deserved to be first.

Nikki's Story

Dear Esteemed Doctors,

What I offer you is my story: five generations of a family affected with cancer. We do not know exactly where the BRCA2 gene mutation originated, but I will share with you what I do know.

My maternal great-grandfather lived a prolific life. He farmed the North Dakota plains to provide a nice life for his wife and twelve children. In 1967, he was diagnosed with breast cancer. Four years later, it took his life. This was a shock to his family and friends, but they had no idea what was in store. Two of his sons and five of his daughters would find themselves in a similar fate. One of those seven children was my grandmother.

Now, I assume most of us do not have a lot of memories at the age of four and five. Studies actually indicate that people have no memories prior to the age of three. My first memories involved my grandmother's struggle with cancer. I have memories as a child, driving with my mother to my grandmother's chemotherapy treatment. I remember seeing her lose her hair, and I was afraid. My mother assured me it was not contagious. How was she to know that we also had the same gene mutation that was proliferating itself throughout our family?

I was five years old when I attended my grandmother's funeral. I remember the devastation on the faces of the seven children and husband that she left behind.

I remember wondering, "Will my mom also die?"

I was afraid.

Four years later, at the young, invincible age of twenty-nine, my grandmother's daughter, my mother's sister, Anna, would hear a diagnosis her mother heard not so long ago: She had breast cancer. Five years later, we buried a beautiful mother of two sons. The pain on the children's faces is something nobody should have to witness.

Now I look back and wonder if the doctor and my aunt had decided against breast-conserving surgery and decided to move forward with a more aggressive approach, would Anna's life and death have been different? But how were they to know their decision would ultimately cost Anna her life?

Two years later, another diagnosis rang throughout the family; another daughter, sister and mother heard the words that were now feared by everyone. My aunt Fran had cancer. After the initial diagnosis, she had her left breast removed and kept her right breast. Five years and six months later, the cancer reoccurred in her other breast. By the time it was detected, it had already spread to her lymph nodes. She fought for four more years before the cancer took her life at the age of forty-two. She left behind two daughters and a son.

Fear and sadness shook the family. Who was going to be next? I was afraid I would lose my mother like my cousins had lost theirs.

I think it is important to note, that from the initial diagnosis to the time of their deaths, the quality of their lives was less than optimal. In both the cases I referenced above, the cancer metastasized to their brains, and they died very long and painful deaths, while their families hopelessly watched.

As I look back, I now realize that a subconscious fear would awaken during certain milestones and moments of my life. I recall going through puberty and developing breasts. While my friends joyously celebrated purchasing their first bras, I wondered if and when my breasts would betray me as they had so many others within my family. By that point in my life, I realized that my mother had been mistaken, breast cancer was contagious, at least within our family, and I was afraid.

When I was nineteen years old, I went for a routine annual physical. The doctor conducting my breast exam found something a bit suspicious. I remember feeling the blood drain from my face. Was it already time for the inevitable to occur? I was afraid.

At the time, I did not realize my mother was experiencing the same fear. Parents typically do not share their own fears with their children.

When my mother was forty-two years old, a suspicious lump was found. She was tired. She was tired of being afraid. Right then and there, she decided that regardless of the results of the suspicious lump, she was going to proceed with a mastectomy. Two doctors refused to operate. Back then, it was considered too radical and too extreme. She was not deterred, only more resilient. She found a surgeon who had recently lost his sister to breast cancer and also had a strong background of breast cancer in his family. Finally, my mother found someone who understood and listened.

Two months later she completed her prophylactic mastectomy with reconstructive surgery. The lump turned out to be benign. It was a wakeup call that my mother gave thanks to. I remember feeling a great sense of relief. I no longer had to feel afraid for my mother. This marked a turning point in my family history.

Ten years later, my mother's doctor referred her to a genetic counselor to explore the possibility of genetic testing. After weeks of dialogue and fact finding, the genetic counselor advised my mother not to test. There were a few reasons given for this recommendation. However, I call it paralysis by the analysis. One of the reasons given was that there is a possibility the gene mutation causing cancer in our family is different from the gene mutation being identified in the test, thus giving a false negative. My response to that: You have not lost anything; you just remain where you are, which is in the world of unknown.

We were fortunate that my mother had complications unrelated to cancer that prompted her to move forward with an oophorectomy.

Over the next ten years, we buried a few more of my mother's aunts to cancer. I proceeded to get married and have a beautiful daughter and the most handsome of sons. My fear shifted; I was now afraid of prematurely leaving my children.

When I was thirty years old, a friend of mine in the healthcare industry told me a bit more about genetic testing and how it was advancing. I was interested in pursuing the testing but where would I start? What does the testing entail?

Dr. Stephen Covey states that it is human nature to focus on the urgent items in our lives[10]. Urgent means it requires immediate attention, now! Urgent matters are usually visible. They press on us. They insist on action. We react to urgent matters.

Important matters, on the other hand, that are not urgent require more initiative. Genetic testing fell into this category. We must act to seize opportunity, to make things happen. Genetic testing was important. However, the urgent things in life were taking a priority (career, kids, husband, etc.). For the next two years, my quest for genetic testing would surface during my annual OB/GYN visit. I would inquire. My OB/GYN would get a confused look on her face and give me a phone number to try. The phone number would ultimately lead me to nowhere and once again the genetic testing would get placed on the back burner.

On my thirty-third birthday, I decided that it was time to make this testing an urgent priority in my life. I had a very real understanding that I would turn thirty-four on my next birthday, the same age that my aunt died of breast cancer. I could no longer delay my quest for knowledge. My friend in the healthcare industry provided me with the name and number of a nurse practitioner who could do the blood test.

Blood test? Is that all there is to it? If it is just a simple blood test why was it so difficult for me to get it done?

Finally, on October 18, 2009, my blood was drawn. On Tuesday, November 14, I received my results. I was BRCA2 positive, and I was no longer afraid. I was no longer afraid, because the unknown was now known. I was empowered with choices! I no longer felt like prey waiting for the inevitable.

I remember sharing the information with my mother. It was a difficult conversation to have. We both cried. My mother cried tears a mother cries when something is wrong with her children and because she knew the mutation gene came from her.

We cried for the people who had passed before us who were not privy to this information. I weighed my options and decided to take a two-stage approach. The first phase was to move forward with a prophylactic mastectomy. The next phase would be to have a prophylactic oophorectomy.

On February 22, 2009, I underwent a prophylactic mastectomy with reconstructive surgery. My mother was there, holding my hand, and I felt so thankful that I still had her in my life for yet another milestone.

A lot of people have asked me if my decision to have the prophylactic mastectomy was difficult. The answer was and is: No, the decision was not difficult. Many women in my family lost their lives to breast cancer. I know that if they had been given the choice to see their children graduate from high school, experience their first loves, get married, and see their grandchildren, they would have done whatever necessary to make that happen. I feel sadness that they did not have the knowledge I so gratefully have.

Now, some of you might be interested in my siblings' response to discovering we have the BRAC2 genetic mutation in our family. I have two brothers. My older brother is your typical single male, resistant to doctors. He has no intention of pursuing the test.

My younger brother, however, has a different perspective. He has children of his own. His initial question was, "If I have the test and test negative will I ever have to have this conversation with my children?"

I told him he would not. He then stated, "I don't go to the doctor much, but the next time I have any blood work done, I will include the test for this genetic mutation."

I informed him it was not that easy. We would have to find somebody in his area who could do the blood test. It should be and needs to be easier. Somebody has to do something. Then I realized that somebody was me and each of you. It is our generation that is going to make the difference in terms of the availability of these tests.

Roughly fifty-six percent of my great-grandfather's children have been afflicted with cancer. It now is affecting the generations of his grandchildren and great grandchildren. The statistics continue to startle me. I recently learned his last remaining son, who is a breast cancer survivor, had four daughters. Every single one of them has had breast cancer. That is one-hundred percent of his children!

I mentioned that my letter to you would demonstrate how this genetic mutation has impacted five generations. Think of how many future generations are going to benefit from this knowledge. You have the ability to make a difference for generations and generations of people who you have identified. I implore you to ask the extra questions to respond to your patient's needs. My children, your children, and your patients' children are going to benefit (or not) from the decisions that you make today.

Teri Smieja

This letter is articulate and compelling! I can feel Nikki's fear turned to strength, and that's the power of having this genetic test performed. I'm grateful to Nikki for taking the time to write her story. I felt, for a few minutes, that I was alongside her in her journey. I am so confused, though, with so many generations of breast cancer, why, oh why, was it so difficult to get a doctor to agree to letting Nikki, or her mother before her, take that test? Like she said, it's just a simple blood test!

This is why I believe *Letters to Doctors* is so important. This letter was written in a way that any doctor, nurse practitioner (NP), or physician's assistant (PA) should be able to read and feel a part of Nikki's life.

Bravo to Nikki for taking real charge of her life, and for taking the steps she took.

Dr. Herman

Thank you, Nikki, for your letter. I had my office staff read it, and I asked them what they learned from it. This is what they had to say:

- *Men get breast cancer. They didn't all know that.*
- *BRCA mutations can pass through the paternal side of the family. They didn't all know that.*
- *Patients want to know why their family members get breast cancer.*
- *Many women from breast and ovarian cancer families are living in fear.*
- *BRCA testing, positive or negative can replace fear with empowerment.*
- *Patients will do what they need to do to avoid getting cancer.*
- *Wow. Some of our patients could get cancer and even die if we don't get this information for them before cancer strikes.*

Voices from the Crowd

We would like to introduce you to Voices from the Crowd. These are comments and quotes from our friends, patients and family members in response to reading these letters. We found they are both educational and interesting.

Katrina W.

Nikki, you did it! You changed the fate of future generations. I'm BRCA2 positive from my grandfather. He was also from North Dakota and it took his only two children. And it is amazing how that blood test will change the lives of my children and their children. They won't have to live with the fear we grew up with. That positive test was one of the best days of my life because I knew what I was fighting.

Sarah K.

Hi, Nikki, why didn't your doctor tell you to get BRCA tested? I think he dropped the ball. You shouldn't have to find out about it on your own. You shouldn't have to be the one to request testing. What happens if someone never heard of BRCA? Should they just get sick?

Letters of Praise

Dr. Herman

When Teri and I began putting this book together, the first wave of letters we received was critical. One might even say hypercritical. We wondered if anyone would want to read an entire *Book of Complaints*. We doubted that.

Then, letters of praise appeared. It's easy for patients to criticize. I think, as practitioners, we listen all day to complaint after complaint. I admit I learned a lot from my patients that were critical of my office and my actions, but throughout the years, the lion's share of letters I have saved are ones that say: Thank you.

Here, we point out some valuable lessons from these letters of praise.

You will notice that the names of some of the practitioners are included in the letters of praise while in the more critical letters, their names are not always included. We decided to include names when a practitioner is praiseworthy, while throughout *Letters to Doctors*, criticized providers have not been identified.

Sarah A.

Dear Professor G, I love you! It is normal, isn't it, to fall for your doctor? I know that you are married, have children, and even grandchildren, and that all your other patients probably love you, but I still love you. You have been there through all the ups and downs (cysts and more cysts and breast cancer cells) of my breast cancer journey since being referred by your colleague from over the ditch.

You were there for twelve hours during my breast reconstruction surgery along with your team that you trust. You listened to me.

You answered my questions. You allowed me to choose what surgery I had. You gave me trust in you without taking away my decision-making power.

You are also there now for my daughter who has had breast cysts since she was seventeen. I know that whatever decisions she has to make in the future (she is also BRCA2 positive) you will be there to give her the same affirmation in her decisions.

Yes, I love you.

Angela L.

Dr. G., I am an ovarian cancer Previvor, thanks to you. I have a predisposition but have not been diagnosed with cancer. Together, we have reduced my odds of getting ovarian cancer. You listened to my thoughts and researched information, gave me your opinion, which was on the same path as mine, and allowed me to make the ultimate decision as to what operation and the time frame in which to have it, mindful of the fact that I shouldn't wait too long.

You were sensitive to my needs at all times, and it may sound old fashioned, but you were a real gentleman, who showed respect for me as a woman. This above all makes you stand out as an exceptional person who deals with BRCA positive women. Thank you.

DeAnna Howe Rice

Because of a doctor who was so committed to treating people, a doctor who wasn't even my doctor, I am here today. You took the time to listen to my story, and you were wise enough to launch on me like a pit bull. To Dr. Lisa Curcio, I owe you my life. Thank you for educating me and all the many people you have reached. It is my honor to call you a friend.

In a sentence, I need to acknowledge the doctors and healthcare professionals who treated me poorly, like a number. Not taking the time to see me as a person, a mom, a wife, a daughter, a sister, a friend. Those of you who made insensitive comments. Those of you who were downright rude and bordered on cruel. I hope no one you know is ever treated the way you treated me.

This is all the time I will waste on you.

Janet B.

Dear Current GP, by the time I began coming to your practice, my life and health journey with breast cancer was a long way down the road. You know I am proactive about treatment and referrals I wish to pursue, and you basically refer me to anyone I need, because you listen to me. You know I do not do things lightly. There is thought, research and positivity in all I do with regard to my life and my health.

The biggest thing you have done was to support me in my request for BRCA testing. This has not only saved me from breast cancer recurrence, but because of this knowledge, I have also been able to reduce my chances of getting ovarian cancer. In agreeing to support me in this testing, you have also had a massive impact on my daughter's life and health, as she has been able to also be tested. Knowing we are BRCA positive is empowering for both me and my daughter. I will be forever grateful for your trust that I know what I am doing with my requests.

You actively listen, respond, and if you are unsure, you are honest. You get back to me once you have done research and share the information in a way that encourages and affirms decisions I must make. I could not ask for anything more in a GP. Thank you.

- *Truly listen to what we have to say.*
- *Try to understand what we think about.*
- *Answer our questions.*
- *We want your opinion.*
- *Treat us with honesty and respect.*
- *Treat us like you would treat your family members if they were in our situation.*
- *When you don't know, it's okay to say so.*
- *Support our desire to be tested.*

Louisa

Dear GP from Twenty-Four Years Ago,

If it wasn't for you, I could well be dead! Yes, I found the lump and acted on it, but you didn't dismiss it. Even though I was only thirty-three, you followed through and sent me to a surgeon you trusted.

It turned out I did have breast cancer and had surgery and treatment. You were stunned to hear the diagnosis, because way back then, women in my age group weren't diagnosed with breast cancer. Everyone I met during my treatment was in their fifties, sixties, and beyond. They had grandchildren my daughter's age. It was a weird experience to go through it back then. You did not blame me like a few others whom I had to deal with during treatment did. You saved my life, and my husband, daughter and I will be forever grateful.

Nina W.

Dear Dr. LaVoe (My Son's Pediatrician),

A few years back, my eldest son had a lump on his neck. I came in and met with you. It ended up being nothing. I had said I always worry about any kind of lump or bump. I then shared that my mother died of ovarian cancer. When you heard this, you started to talk to me about genetic testing. I said, "I know. I just don't know if I want to know."

You looked me in the eye and said, "Do it for your kids."

Wow! You hit home. I had just begun to research the idea. It was all still foreign to me. I tucked this information away with other info I had gathered along my journey.

Dr. LaVoe, I did hear you. Later that year, I decided to do BRCA testing. Turns out I am BRCA1 positive. I had risk-reducing surgery and plan to live a long healthy life!

Thanks for sharing your knowledge with me.

~~Dr. Ira LaVoe. DO, FACOP, special interests include general pe-
diatrics, early childhood development, learning disabilities, and
pediatric emergency medicine. He is a member of Broomall Pediatric
Associates in Broomall, PA.

L.

Dear Dr. F. (Plastic Surgeon),

Thank you for suggesting to my sister she have the BRCA
screening 1997, over a year after she had been found to have
peri-menopausal breast cancer at age fifty-two. After her cancer was discovered in one breast, she chose bilateral
mastectomies with tram flaps as she did not want to worry
about breast cancer in the other breast as well. We didn't have
much cancer history in our family, but we are of Ashkenazi
Jewish descent. You were thinking properly and had my sister
tested!

When her test came back positive, my sister, of course, called
me immediately, suggesting I get tested. We both had excellent guidance and support for the testing by a genetic
counseling team, but it was all new back then. When my results were positive, the team assembled to meet me and
answer my questions. A geneticist, a pathologist, and an advanced practice nurse were all in the room, and my very new
husband was with me to ask questions and give me support.

My sister died of metastatic breast cancer in 2010, sixteen years
after her initial diagnosis. Maybe, just maybe you (and she)
saved my life. You did my preventive mastectomies in 1999,
and I am healthy!

Thank you, Dr. F. I will never forget you!

Lisa Grocott

Dr. Constance Chen (Plastic Surgeon),

I only write references at the request of my graduate students, so I am not in the habit of writing unsolicited references. But it is easy to be motivated to write when the person you are commending is someone you know you will always feel indebted to.

When I found out I was BRAC2 positive, I began to research which type of prophylactic surgery to have. Once I had decided to have the DIEP procedure, I went on to research surgeons. I was based in New York, and I was confident I could have the best of the best. I found the surgeon in town who was the most highly recommended, whose office was super professional, and who had been doing this procedure longer than anyone else. I was sure I had found my surgeon. I next heard that he couldn't take my insurance and, although initially devastated, I quickly came to see that this was my lucky break, because the practice then recommended the wonderful Dr. Chen to me. Knowing what I know now about what makes a surgeon great, I look back on my early decision-making and my criteria for selecting a surgeon seems so misplaced.

From the first day, Dr. Chen became my primary surgeon; she also became my advocate with the surgical team. With Dr. Chen, I always knew someone was in my corner. With the initial surgery, she challenged the surgical team to try a nipple-sparing mastectomy on hilariously large breasts, and in the reconstructive surgery, she encouraged her surgical partner to spend an extra hour to really make things perfect. This combination of perfectionism, ambition, and dedication all translated to me being incredibly happy with the results and feeling like I really did get the best of the best. And for all this, I will be eternally grateful.

But at the end of the day, what I will really remember about Dr. Chen and her team is how they helped to make a really sucky time in my life seem okay. Her staff was always amazing. They were professional and efficient, but more importantly, they were empathetic and thoughtful. The single image that will stick in my mind is Dr. Chen's smiling face each time I came out of surgery. She'd be standing over me with the most inane grin, buzzing with enthusiasm for how well the surgery went. I knew then, even in a drugged haze, that she loved her job and really cared about each individual patient.

I couldn't help but wonder a few times over the eighteen months I was in Dr. Chen's care whether the fact she was a female surgeon made a difference. I am certain there are male surgeons out there as equally talented as she, but I am not so confident that as many of them would realize that just sitting with your patient for two hours on a Friday night in hospital might be just what your patient needs.

I am pleased Dr. Chen is so dedicated, because it meant she replied to my weekend emails. I am glad I found a plastic surgeon who is such a perfectionist, because I now have breasts ten times more beautiful than they were before. I am glad she was ambitious, because I got to keep my own nipples, even when it had never been done on breasts my size before. But above all, I am grateful I found a surgeon who is compassionate and a good listener, because that meant I never felt alone or scared.

~~*Dr. Constance M. Chen is a board-certified plastic surgeon who specializes in complex microsurgical breast reconstruction. She operates at Lenox Hill Hospital[11], and the New York Eye and Ear Infirmary[12] as part of the New York Center for the Advancement of Breast Reconstruction[13].*

Recap

- *Keep the lines of communication open.*
- *Become our advocate.*
- *This is stressful. Often, we can't remember what you told us. Sending a summary or calling the next day does wonders!*
- *We would like the option of being introduced to other patients when possible.*
- *We oftentimes don't mind sharing our stories with your patients; ask us if we'd be willing.*
- *We may love you, but your staff sometimes could do a lot better.*

Voices from the Crowd

Raechel Maki

Both my sister and I are BRCA1 positive. We know that, thanks to our outstanding family physician, who took the time to care about us, we both owe our lives to her. To ignore the precious gift of knowledge we have been given would be like kicking my mother in the face and spitting on her fight and hope to live.

Lisa Grocott

I have had so many positive experiences with medical professionals, it is hard to think of what they did that worked so well. I liked how my GYN/ONC was extremely up to date with her research and excellent at providing her advice on what I should do.

Lily

If I had to pick the one thing out of all the positive experiences I have had, it would be the fact that my doctor put his pen on the table and turned off his computer and said, "Let me hear what you are thinking." That's it.

I Am BRCA Positive

Dr. Herman

In this section, Teri and I wanted to capture some of the intense feelings of those who tested positive for BRCA mutations. BRCA positive women (and men) have very valid but divergent ideas about treatment options, surveillance, prophylactic surgery, breast reconstruction, relationships, children, childrearing and careers, just to list a few. In the early days of genetic testing, I think that there was a general belief that women couldn't handle a positive result. I know that's not true. It didn't take long to learn that these ladies are tough as nails.

Teri Smieja

When I first heard that the BRCA1 mutation ran in my family (mom's side), I knew immediately that I would be tested for it. I didn't go through the process of trying to decide if I should be tested or not. I didn't for even one moment consider not finding out if my BRCA1 gene was mutated. I *had* to know.

During the time I spent waiting for my test results, I tried to comfort myself with the awareness that if I did end up having the mutation, at least there were things I could do about it. Having the mutation did not have to mean an automatic death sentence for me as it had for some of my family.

Janice M.

Dear Dr. Herman,

I just listened to your lecture on HBOC. I found it very informative. Thank you. I have spent more than a year trying to get my BRCA genes tested. After being turned down twice by my insurance for not having enough relatives with the disease, I appealed, won my appeal, and had genetic counseling done.

I was informed today that I am positive for the gene mutation. After listening to your lecture[14], I wonder if I also carry Lynch Syndrome. My maternal great grandmother died of uterine cancer in her late thirties or early forties.

Thank you for your explanation of testing family and plans for health surveillance. I plan to mail my genetic report and my BRCA report to each of my sisters in the morning. I remember learning years ago about ovarian and breast cancer being on the same gene, and now we have advanced enough scientifically to look for it.

Thank you again, and God bless!

Getting Tested Should Be Easy

Teri's Blog

It took fifty-two days, one improperly carried out test, and finally, a correctly-performed test for me to obtain my BRCA test results.

I'll never forget that day.

I received a call from one of the staff at my gynecologist's office where I'd had the test done. The receptionist told me over the phone that I had tested positive for BRCA1. I had the breast cancer gene mutation. I felt like a zombie. My eyes filled with tears while I contemplated what this meant to me and to my family. What would be my next step? What would happen? What should I do? Was I going to die an early death?

I asked my eldest son, Steven, to come with me to the doctor's office so he could wait in the car with my baby, Brady, while I ran in to pick up my test results.

I pulled up outside the office, went in, and the receptionist handed me the report. She smiled at me, reassuringly, and told me they had the name of an oncologist they could refer me to if I was interested. That was about it. I didn't actually get the name of the doctor though. Through my scared and confused haze, I forgot to ask. She had a sympathetic smile plastered on her face when she shifted uncomfortably in her chair. "Was that it?" she flatly asked.

I wondered, *Do I just take the results from her and leave?*

In many ways, I felt like I had been given a diagnosis of cancer rather than the diagnosis of a predisposition to cancer. The fear that I'd been obsessing over those past fifty-two days had just become a reality. My local gynecologist's office had never dealt with this sort of thing before, this BRCA mutation. They had no plan on what to do next. It really wasn't their forte. I was on my own to figure out the next steps.

I thanked her, which on hindsight seems odd, and I numbly walked back to the car while I tried to process my test results. I had the BRCA1 mutation, passed onto me from my mother and to her from hers. Where it came from before that is any-one's guess.

While I didn't recall knowledge of the BRCA mutation up until the point I was told I should test for it, I did have an inkling that I was prone to ovarian cancer as a few of my relatives had it. I had never thought about it as it applied to me. I had never thought about my own mortality because of it. In fact, I used to smoke about a half pack of cigarettes per day, and I never spent much time thinking I might get cancer from it and die. So why, all of a sudden, when I got confirmation that I had the mutation, were thoughts of my death taking over my mind?

I tried to blink away the tears, only to find my face staring back at me in the rearview mirror. My son's eyes were wide while he watched me, not sure what to do. I met his gaze and more tears poured. I thought how terrible it would be to die without seeing my teenager and baby become men. In just a few moments, so many thoughts convoluted my thinking. I wondered how my husband would raise the baby, alone, without me. The whole drive home I thought about it. I thought of my funeral, and wondered how much it would hurt to die of breast or ovarian cancer.

Now, a few years down the line from that day, you might wonder how I'm doing now. Well, the thing is, BRCA is still a part of my life. My BRCA diagnosis changed me forever. It changed me in a way that I'm very proud of. I feel I took a horrible, deadly hand and turned it into a royal flush.

Practitioner's Question

Dr. Herman, how do you handle telling someone they are positive?

Dr. Herman

Early on, I used to get flustered (just read Teri's letter above). Initially, I was worried about how to go about discussing results. I wasn't sure I would be able to deal properly with the reactions. However, experience makes for a good teacher, and boy, did I learn.

One of the foremost lessons I learned is to make myself available immediately and on an ongoing basis to these patients. I use my office hours to contact BRCA positive patients. Most of the time, that means calling them at 7:30 in the morning and catching them before I start my day. I make sure my staff is aware the patient is coming in, to minimize any delay in the waiting room. I also remind them the patient will be in crisis mode. Whatever time is needed, the patient is entitled to it, and they get it no matter how busy the office is that day. If another patient complains that they had to wait because I took too long, I just tell them, "You don't want to have what the last patient has." That works.

Oftentimes, I start the appointment with a warm greeting and quick hug. It seems to put my patients at ease, and it lets them know I'm here for them. When we sit down, I review all the information that was given at the time of the genetic counseling visit. I always go over the numbers, but find the general concepts are what the patients remember. I give a results handout with the statistics so it can be reviewed later, once they've had some time to think about what it means to be BRCA positive.

How much does the patient remember from this visit? Almost nothing. Most patients can't process what I say after the initial minute. Digesting the gravity of the situation takes longer, often days, months, or even years. It's not that the patients are not intelligent or have an inability to handle the implications. Simply put, when in crisis mode, most people can't process that many inputs in such a short span of time.

- *Meet with your patients.*
- *Prepare your staff.*
- *Give your patients the time they need.*
- *Handouts are very helpful.*
- *Give your patients copies of their test results.*

Laura R.
I Couldn't Believe It!

I had just gotten home from working a graveyard shift and had been asleep about an hour or two when my doctor called. I swear I thought it was a nightmare I was having. I just kept saying, "I can't believe it."

My sweet doctor stayed on the phone with me while I tried to wake up and accept what I heard. I was in complete shock and my husband couldn't believe it either. My first fear was for my children. My husband and I saw my doctor later that day and we went over my options. For weeks, I couldn't bear to be alone, because my mind went to a really dark place.

Today, I am actually doing great. After having both prophylactic surgeries, I have gone from being scared and sad to feeling strong and empowered. That is due, I believe, to the wonderful doctors I have had and incredible online support groups, like the BRCA Sisterhood!

Dr. Herman

You may wonder what else happens when I sit down with my patients. In addition to the handout, I like to empower the person who has accompanied the patient. That applies to all visits going forward. For every important doctor's visit, I encourage my patients to bring a spouse, relative, or a friend. On the first visit, I remind everyone present that there is so much to absorb and remember, it's nearly impossible to do it in the span of one visit. I encourage my patients and/or their support person to take notes and start a folder to keep track of all BRCA-related information. I tell them, "Get one of those marble composition notebooks like you had in elementary school." Months later, many have come back to tell me that it was the best tip they received.

The initial visit is just that, an *initial* visit. It is the beginning of the journey. Taking care of BRCA positive families is a dynamic and an ongoing process. It must be viewed that way. It requires an integrated approach to care. Involved in the follow up are the mammographers, breast MRI specialists, breast surgeons, medical oncologists, gynecologists, GYN/ONCs, genetic counselors, and psychologists, to name a few. For my patients, I've put together a list of practitioners I recommend, with their names and numbers that I hand out. This type of handout has worked out well.

I always try to guide my patients. I let them know which doctors to see next and what's to follow. I suggest alternatives so that if doctor A can't see them or doesn't take their insurance plan, they'll have another option. In my opinion, just handing these patients a list and calling it a day isn't good enough. The list has to come with some information about each practitioner. This establishes a necessary comfort level between the new physician and patient. The radiologist I send most of my patients to is one I have been working with the past ten plus years. I make sure the patients know my wife goes to him for her mammography. It provides a level of comfort for my patients. The patient knows, "This is where Dr. Herman's wife goes for her mammograms."

It bothers me to hear that a patient found a surgeon from one of her coworkers or from her aunt's daughter's boyfriend's mother. This is not the time to send a patient on a discovery mission or wild goose chase to find out who is the best.

Review the reason you are sending your patient for each visit and what she will need for that visit. No one wants to waste time. For example, prior to scheduling an appointment with the radiologist, let her know to have all of her old films, x-rays, or MRI reports available for the doctor. If not, her visit will be suboptimal.

I give my patients many copies of their BRCA report, because I insist they give one to every physician they see. If they have had an important study dealing with HBOC, I make sure to put a copy of the report in their hands, too.

Keep in mind: I try to have an open-door policy, and I make sure all of my patients are made aware of it. Any time, they can call me, and I will fit them in. The day the patient receives her test results will only be the first of the crisis days.

Let's return to the initial visit: At the end of the appointment, the patient can't wait to leave. What happens next? I have seen it time and time again. She goes out to the car, sits in the parking lot, and cries for a half hour. Forget going to work.

After getting home, she bounces around the house for a couple of hours and then sits down at the computer. By evening, she's had some time to collect her thoughts and think through some of her decisions. I make it my business to call that night. You will discover how valuable that call is as the patient remembers more from that call than from her office visit earlier in the day.

Most practitioners have strong feelings on what the plan of care should be when they receive their patient's positive BRCA results from the lab. I know I do. The patient might have a very different view. We must be overly sensitive to the way we provide this critical information to each patient so that it encourages the best medical management decisions. For that patient, the follow up will depend on her individual needs.

- *Provide for effective discussion so that your patient can make informed medical decisions.*
- *Suggest that your patient record each visit's highlights in a notebook.*
- *Suggest that your patient bring a support person with her to each visit.*
- *Review the cancer risks associated with a positive result.*

- *Review medical management options with the patient.*
- *Discuss the importance of sharing test results with their first-degree relatives.*
- *Provide multiple copies of the test results and the patient results brochure to the patient.*
- *Offer information about support groups.*
- *Ensure a regular schedule of follow-up visits.*
- *Be available and accessible.*

Sara K.
The Shock Came After

I didn't tell my family I was being tested because I knew what I would do if I was positive. So I was alone when I went to get my results, and I was not shocked when I heard her tell me I was positive. For me, the shock came afterward.

The counselor was explaining the screening and telling me that I did not need to consider anything other than screening until I was forty. I told her I wanted to be connected with the doctor who would do a mastectomy. She seemed so surprised that, at twenty-nine, I would be so willing to go that route right away. She tried to tell me that she thought I didn't need to do this so early; I pointed at my family cancer tree my aunt had made for us, and told her I was not taking any chances.

Katrina W.
I Started to Cry

The day I found out I was BRCA positive, I was at home with my girls when the genetic counselor called. I remember her saying I was positive, and I started to cry. It was such a relief. I know it sounds crazy, but I wanted that test to be positive so badly for myself, for my cousin, for my mother I had lost, for her mother she had lost, for my daughters. I was happy we finally had an answer. It was empowering, because I could now do something to save myself, my family, and my girls. It was also sad learning who the killer was a little too late, and having to call family and tell them you finally have the answer, just too late (for some family members). Funny, out of all the emotions since that day, fear has never been one of them. I'm not afraid.

Dr. Herman

My very first BRCA-positive patient was diagnosed on June 25, 2006.

I entered the hospital and made my way down the main corridor, took a quick left, and then went up two flights of stairs. I used my ID card to get onto the labor and delivery floor (L&D). When I swung the door open, Jennifer, one of our L&D nurses, was standing in the doorway. She said hello and asked if I knew where she could go for BRCA testing. Proud of the fact I had been counseling patients, I told her I would take care of everything. During her break, I sat with her in the nurse's lounge for an hour.

I had no clue that, as a teenager, she had lost her mother to breast cancer and that her grandmother brought her up along with her two sisters. Neither was I aware her maternal aunt, her mother's sister, had been diagnosed with breast cancer. For over a decade, we worked together, but I never knew this aspect of her life. Ten days later, her results arrived via FedEx. As I looked inside the envelope, I felt sick to see that Jen's results were positive for a deleterious mutation. This was the first positive test result I had ever had. Over the next few years, Jennifer would always remind me with a big smile that she was my first.

I must have made twenty calls before I contacted her. I spoke with a genetic counselor, another GYN/ONC, mammographer, breast surgeon, plastic surgeon, my wife, my partners, and a few other trusted colleagues in order to make sure I didn't miss any aspect of dealing with a positive result. I spoke with Jen and together we started working on a treatment plan.

We agreed to keep it quiet. Two things began to happen the very next day. The first, almost every nurse on staff asked me how Jen was handling the news. So much for keeping it quiet. Second, for the next few weeks after I would finish up a delivery, hospital employees would meet me at the delivery room door wanting to tell me their personal cancer family history. They weren't my patients. Why hadn't their physicians taken care of this? Why was it that Jennifer had to go looking for someone to get this testing done? It also occurred to me that medical personnel are exceptions. The typical patient doesn't request testing.

Many had never even heard of BRCA. As a doctor, I had better be prepared to identify those in need.

Nicki W.
I Knew I Was Positive

I felt like I already knew I was positive. The doctor opened the envelope in front of me and said, "It's positive."

My response was, "I know."

I had never allowed myself to believe it would come back negative. It was a very surreal day, and I don't think it sank in what the results meant until a few days later.

Teri's Blog

I have to say that sometimes I feel guilty, too. I feel guilty that I have the opportunity to have prophylactic (preventative or risk-reducing) surgeries when so many others didn't get that chance. So many women have lost their breasts, their ovaries, their lives to breast or ovarian cancer. A few men with the BRCA mutation have battled breast cancer, too (dispel the myth, men do get breast cancer). If only they had known of their BRCA mutation before they got the cancer, then they could be sitting where I am, with months to research, time to think about their choices, a chance to meet other women who have gone through it. But they didn't have that chance.

They were thrown into a dark hole of cancer, fear, and despair, and their choices had to be made quickly. Treatments had to start immediately. Most times, body parts had to be removed. Sometimes parts should have been removed but weren't. Some battled and won. Some lost.

After reading other blogs about cancer, my feelings of guilt are strong. I can't help but wonder if any of those women met me, if they wouldn't like to just come over and slap my face at the injustice of it. How I wish they had known before the cancer struck. I wish they had the same chance that I am getting.

Dr. Herman

I spoke in Rochester, New York, on August 14, 2012, and NP and MD from the same office were interested to hear more about the day they found out they were BRCA positive.

I shared Samantha's story with them.

Samantha Skyler
I Was Tested When Pregnant

My childhood was anything but normal. When I was eleven years old and my sister, Heather, was seven, my mother, Francine, was diagnosed with breast cancer. I really wasn't sure what that meant, but for the next two years, I watched her go through surgeries and many treatments that made her sick and changed her personality.

When I was thirteen, she passed away in the hospital. She was thirty-six years old. It wasn't until that time that I learned about my family history. My grandmother, Cecilia, and my Aunt Judith both had breast cancer but were lucky enough to have survived.

My father spent the next several years researching and reading up on the newest treatments and preventative measures on the market for breast cancer. He casually suggested my sister and I consider going to Sloane Kettering to participate in a study. The study was focused on children who had lost a mother to breast cancer. My sister and I didn't immediately pursue it, because at the time, I was fourteen years old and she was ten. It seemed like something that happened to our mother would never happen to us.

After my mother's death, many things happened in my life. I finished high school, graduated with a bachelor's degree from college and attended graduate school, where I received my Masters of Social Work (MSW).

I met my husband when I was twenty-seven years old. We got engaged and married and began planning a family. In between all of this, I went for yearly mammograms and sonograms and held my breath until the results came. I was so thankful every year that went by that I had no signs of lumps in my breasts.

Samantha's Family Red Flags

Mother	breast cancer
Maternal side aunt	breast cancer
Maternal side aunt	breast cancer
Ethnic Background	Ashkenazi Jewish Ancestry

In March 2006, my husband and I were ecstatic when we found out I was pregnant. My obstetrician was Dr. Herman.

During my first visit with him, he asked about my family history and came to realize I had a strong history of breast cancer in my family. Dr. Herman discussed with me the idea of BRCA testing after pregnancy. I was hesitant. After careful thought, I realized I wanted to take the test for my future children. I felt responsible to know if I carry the mutation and the likelihood of passing it down.

I initially felt that if I tested positive, there was nothing I could do except wait. Dr. Herman reassured me that there were options. I chose to find out during my pregnancy.

As expected, I tested positive for the BRCA2 mutation. I say expected, but it was still extremely difficult to know for sure that I was at such high risk for breast cancer. After much discussion with my wonderful husband and Dr. Herman, I decided to have the prophylactic surgery done after my son was born, once I'd finished breastfeeding him.

My son was born in November 2006, and I met with plastic surgeons and breast doctors during my maternity leave from work. All confirmed I was making the right choice. That was important to me. On December 21, 2007, I had a double mastectomy and my breast reconstruction was done on March 19, 2008.

I look back on both those surgeries, and I feel lucky I went through them. I took control of something that made me feel so out of control for so many years.

When I wrote this, my son was almost two years old. And the plan was that, after the birth of our second child, I would have my ovaries removed.

My goal in life is to walk my son down the aisle at his wedding and grow old with my husband. These are things my mother never got to do, and I want to do this in her honor.

P.S. I wish she knew she saved my life. Maybe she does.

- *Take a family history on every patient at every yearly visit (things change, updated info is crucial).*
- *That includes your pregnant patients.*
- *Your patients at risk for HBOC may decide to test even while pregnant.*

Patient History

Born 1976

Patient: *Samantha Skyler*

Age 11	Mother, breast cancer at age 34
Age 13	Mother, dies at age 36
Age 24	Begins mammograms & ultrasounds
Age 28	Gets married
Age 30	Pregnancy
Age 30	March, prenatal visit, identifies at risk of HBOC, tests positive
Age 31	November, welcomes a son, breastfeeds
Age 32	December, undergoes risk-reducing mastectomy
Age 32	March, reconstruction complete
Age 32	January, pregnant again
Age 32	Sister, Heather, tests negative
Age 33	October, welcomes a daughter
2013	Risk-reducing BSO

- *Women who test positive often feel like they have gained control.*
- *Parents often discuss their BRCA results with their young children.*
- *Parents should explain the issues at a time and level appropriate for the specific child – "The right time."*
- *You, as the health care practitioner, should be there to guide her through the process.*

Teri Smieja

It should be noted again that not only females get, carry or pass on and suffer from the BRCA mutation. The BRCA mutation is *not* gender specific.

Mary B.
The Day I Almost Found Out

The day I almost found out I was BRCA positive, I was in Utah visiting my twin sister, just two months after she found out she had breast cancer and was BRCA positive. I had gotten my blood work drawn just a couple of days before flying from New York to Utah, and when the number for my primary care doctor showed up on caller ID, I froze.

It's too soon to find out, I thought. I don't want to know yet.

But I answered the call only to find out that my blood sample could not be processed until I filled out a form from Myriad Labs. Having just read an informational book my sister had left out for me to find, I knew that Myriad Labs was the only place my blood would be sent and that the lab is in Salt Lake City. So my doctor called the lab and they agreed that I could drop by and complete the paperwork there.

It turned out to be a semi-traumatic event for both my sister and myself as I associated Myriad Labs with BRCA and just didn't want to be there. All that was running through my own mind was, "This is a bad omen."

The woman who assisted me at Myriad was so kind and gentle; it made the process so much easier for me.

When the report did come in, my doctor called and left me a message, then I called back and left her a message, then I carried my cell around all day and ducked into the trash room on a med/surg unit when her next call came. My doctor told me that she had my results back and wanted me to come in as soon as possible to discuss them. I thought, *I'm not f---ing dumb. I know what that means.*

I spoke with my supervisor, just two weeks into my new position, and told her about the call. It was not a huge surprise, as I had mentioned something about BRCA during my job interview. (That's me. I can never keep my mouth shut.)

The next day, I took a friend along to my appointment. My doctor broke the news to me. She had a copy of the standards of care for me (which I had Googled and brought along, also). The rest of my diagnosis day is a blur. I did go to work. I did call the OB/GYN. I don't remember telling my twin sister or my other sisters of the diagnosis. I don't remember telling my friends. But it all unfolded somehow and three months later, I had my BSO and then a few months later my PBM. Now I am coming up on three years since the BSO, have four tattoos to commemorate the journey, and remain cancer free. Knowledge is power.

Stacey R.
My Story: A Whirlwind of Emotion

Dear Doctors, I was hesitant to write my story for various reasons. However, I have to look beyond myself, because this is an opportunity to do something for you. So here is my story:

The few days have been a whirlwind of emotion following the phone call late afternoon Monday with my doctor confirming that I indeed tested positive with the broken BRCA gene.

My husband and I have been living in slow motion. How do you react to finding out such a thing?

"I'm positive?" I asked. I turned to my husband and shook my head in acknowledgement.

"I am positive," this time repeating the words in the affirmative.

My husband was waiting there with me when I got my results. He was also hoping to breathe that anticipated sigh of relief. Hoping the words of the doctor would be, "Stacey, the test was negative."

But those were not the words that reverberated in my ear.

I asked the doctor almost mechanically, "Okay, so now what?"

"I am still at my office. Come with your husband now so we can talk. I can help."

"Fine, we'll be right over," I responded, feeling somewhat numb.

Come over now, I questioned in my mind. *What about reality? That slight glitch called 'the kids'? How will I get a babysitter on such short notice to watch my two little ones?*

"Call your mother," my husband suggested.

"I can't call Mom. She'll ask me why I'm crying. Okay, let me get myself together. I can't cry. I can't cry."

It's been four days now since I found out this news. Honestly, at times I feel sad. Thank G-d I have been healthy all my life. I now realize that I could be walking around with a ticking time bomb inside of me. I can't get sick. I'm young. My children are young, and they need me. I sometimes feel anxious. And sometimes, I feel strong. I need to take charge of this as best I can. I have to eat healthy. I need to exercise. Perhaps, I'll even get into some of that holistic stuff.

I know that most of all, what will help me pull through all this, is prayer. I need to pray.

G-d, help me be healthy. I want to care for my husband and my children and I want to have more children. You have given me such a special job that I don't always appreciate as much as I should. And G-d, I do see that this truly is a blessing. I have a greater risk, a silent potential that lay dormant, and now, I can, with G-d's help, attempt to do something about it.

Now I know more about what my future could bring and hope to take the necessary precautionary measures to protect myself and my family.

- *When receiving positive BRCA results one should initially expect a host of strong emotions that may include anxiety, fear, anger and depression.*
- *Telling a friend about BRCA and HBOC may save their life and the lives of the extended family.*
- *BRCA testing, positive or negative, replaces fear with empowerment.*

DeAnna Howe Rice
My Test Results Are In

I was called in for my results. Dr. Curcio looked at me and told me I was definitely BRCA1 positive. I finally had answers. My cancers were not from something I did wrong, nor was I being punished at all. This was science, genetics.

I swear the angels were singing and my grandma was smiling down at me.

Then the reality of what this diagnosis meant started to be further discussed: prophylactic removal of my fallopian tubes and ovaries and prophylactic double mastectomies and reconstruction if I opted for that. I was in! I would do anything I needed to do to make sure I never had to be diagnosed with cancer again.

I opted for a full hysterectomy. Frankly, if I didn't need it and it had potential to harbor these cancer cells, it had to go!

Voices from the Crowd

Lulu Luke
Cancer Versus Cancer Mutation

In some ways, for many people with cancer who found out they were gene mutation carriers afterwards, it's like a relief. It explains why they got breast cancers at thirty-seven

Alana D.
My Boss Didn't Understand

When I received my diagnosis, I started seeing different doctors to arrange surgeries and learn more about BRCA1. My boss at work did not understand and made comments like I was getting a "free boob job" and "Hey, you won't have your period anymore, lucky you." I was reprimanded for the time I took away from work to see the doctors and was threatened with reduced pay. At one point, I had to say that I would give anything not to be going through this and would she (my boss) like to trade places with me? The answer was no.

Lulu Luke
On the Initial Shock

People who have the mutation, but not cancer, after the initial shock of being a mutation carrier, are interested in screening and preventative surgery and risks to other family members. However, people who had cancer are worried about the actual cancer more. Will it come back? What are the side effects from chemo? How long do I have to wait after my mastectomy to get a contralateral mastectomy and reconstruction? Is triple negative worse than her BRCA2 cancer?

Lee W.
Calm and Prepared

I already knew my mom was positive. I just went in to the doctor's office, and she told me I was BRCA1 positive. I think I was pretty calm and prepared for that answer, but there might have been a hint of nervousness or, "Okay, now what do I do?"

She discussed my options of increased surveillance, surgery, hormones, as well as that I should think about having kids soon. I was only twenty-two or twenty-three at the time, newly married.

Jean H.
No Surprise

I went into my gyn's office and met with the physician's assistant, Michelle. She told me I was BRCA1 positive. I really was not surprised, because I really suspected I was positive. I had a sense of relief to learn that my breast cancer at age forty was caused by something genetic, not from something I did or did not do.

My first concern was that of my sisters. I knew I had to share this information with them as soon as possible. I am one of five girls.

Pat Martin
I Already Knew

I really didn't feel nervous until a couple of days before going in to get the results. That morning, I woke and as soon as I opened my eyes, I just knew I was positive. I even told my husband. Once we got there and the counselor read us the news, she handed me a tissue, and I just looked at her and told her I already knew. She had thought I would be shocked.

My (big) fear was for my children. I held up well until we were waiting for the elevators and then I felt tears running down my face. My husband just held me and told me to go ahead and cry.

Michelle M.
The Day I Found Out

My husband came with me to the appointment. All the way in the car, we were talking about going to celebrate that I was going to be clean and have nothing to worry about. I was not going to have to face breast cancer or ovarian cancer. The odds were with me right? I have three sisters, and two of them already have the BRCA2 mutation, so the odds are that I would not. Fifty/fifty, right?

When we got to the hospital, I remember getting nervous and my husband just squeezing my hand as we got into the elevator. When we reached the office, I remember the counselor opening the door to the waiting room and telling us she would be with us in a few minutes. I saw a look on her face, and I knew the news was not going to be good.

I went into the room and met with the counselor and the doctor. They told me I was positive for the mutation. I told myself I was not going to cry, but the tears came welling up and rolling down my cheek.

Dr. Rubenstien was giving me the statistics and telling me that this was a good thing to know so I could be monitored more closely. After that, it all went fuzzy. All I was thinking about the entire time was if I was going to have enough time to have a baby before I developed cancer, and if I was going to be able to nurse my child. I was only thirty-two. I should not have put my career before starting a family and now I didn't know if the time bomb would go off before I was able to.

When we left the doctor's office, I was crying in the car while my husband drove. I told him I just wanted to go home.

After we were in the car for about ten minutes, my cell phone rang. It was my sister, who is also BRCA2 positive. I had to tell her I had the mutation, too. When she got her BRCA news, she called me, and I told her that it was not a death sentence and that she did not have cancer. Now, she was telling me the same thing. We just cried on the phone together for several minutes.

About thirty minutes into the ride home (rush hour in Chicago), I looked at my husband and told him that I wanted to go out to eat. I told him I wanted to have a "F-U" to cancer dinner. We went to one of our favorite steak houses and had an awesome meal.

We ordered an expensive bottle of wine. Our waiter asked my husband if we were celebrating anything. I teared up and had to look away. My husband then smiled at me and then told the waiter we were celebrating the fact that I am alive.

I always will remember that day.

That was almost two and a half years ago. I now have a one-year-old I just stopped nursing, and I'm getting ready to try for a second child. I am in the monitoring stage, not quite ready for the surgeries yet.

Who Should Be Tested?

Dr. Herman

"Who should be tested? Who should be tested?"

Not a day goes by that I don't hear that question multiple times. Next are many ideas that will help you in practice. Of course, each patient's story should be evaluated on its own merits.

Stacey Axelrad
New York, September 11, 2012

Dear Dr. Herman,

Hey! It's Stacey. My stepmother was just diagnosed with stage III ovarian cancer. She had surgery yesterday and is starting chemo ASAP. Should she think about having the BRCA test?

New York, September 12, 2012

Dear Dr. Herman,

I went to see my stepmother today. They couldn't get all the cancer. It's spread to her lungs, part of her stomach and they believe her liver. While I was there, the doctor came in and we spoke to him about the BRCA test. He didn't feel it was necessary based on family history. I told him that it could help future generations in her family to know, and I brought up clinical trials and PARP inhibitors that could help my step mom. He basically tried to blow me off.

She is going to insist on having the test. I'll let you know what happens. Thank you for your time and advice.

Question from Physician in Houston, Texas:

Dear Dr. Herman,

I really don't see too many patients in my office who should have BRCA testing. Can you review for me who you would test? I thought only patients with cancer should be tested but that doesn't seem right.

Dr. Herman

Great questions! Hereditary screening is indicated in families that have a strong history of breast and/or ovarian cancer. BRCA testing is not utilized for general population screening. An attempt should always be made to test the affected family member, the patient who has cancer. It's the most cost-effective way to test.

For example, a PARA 7 with breast and ovarian cancer who tests negative negates testing her seven children. However, if the patient with cancer is unavailable to test, testing may be indicated for each one of her kids. You understand that a negative result in an unaffected patient doesn't tell us the status of the other siblings. As a general rule we always try to test the person with cancer. However, it is unfortunately too common that the affected member is not readily available.

Kay E.

My story is that it took ten years after six breast-cancer-related family deaths to get an appointment for genetic testing. When I did get the genetic appointment, I was told I couldn't be tested because all the women in the family who had had breast cancer were dead, and they needed a live comparison.

Teri to Kay

Kay, you should have been tested much earlier and never been turned down. I agree. It saddens me how often I hear about this happening.

Dr. Herman
On Being Asked

"Do doctors recommend testing for everyone?"

We are aware there are no tests in medicine ordered for everyone. Pap smears are performed on five-year-olds, and a mammography is not typically performed on ten-year-olds. You can't get an MRI of your brain just because you want one. Insurance won't pay for it. Likewise, BRCA testing isn't offered to everyone. The criteria are based on red flags.

The American Society of Clinical Oncology[15] recommends

"genetic testing be offered when an individual has a personal or family history that suggests a genetic cancer susceptibility and the test can be adequately interpreted and its results will influence diagnosis or management of the patient or family members at risk for hereditary cancer."[16]

Teri

It may reassure you to know that genetic mutations only account for about five to ten percent of breast cancer today. I sometimes feel like I've met all of the other BRCA mutants in the world and hang out with them on Facebook or in the blogosphere all day.

While it does seem like I know a large amount of mutant women, so many more women carry the mutation and have no idea that they do.

I've pieced together that there are usually certain factors that would make one consider having the genetic test done. Some of those factors are:

- *The obvious: someone in the family has tested positive for the BRCA1 or BRCA2 mutation.*
- *A family history of breast cancer. In my personal experience, I can say this isn't always a good indicator; while statistically, I'm at high risk of breast cancer, no one in my family, that I'm aware of, has ever had breast cancer. The closest anyone, to my knowledge, has come to it is my Aunt Lita, who had a prophylactic bilateral mastectomy (PBM). She had surgery to remove what she thought were her healthy breasts to avoid the Big C. Her pathology report came back showing she was pre-cancerous. Had she not had the PBM, she'd no*

doubt be having chemo right now instead of being in the final stages of reconstruction.

She was 68 at the time of PBM and breast cancer just now started to show up. Ovarian cancer has been more prevalent in my family than breast cancer, so far.

That news didn't make me feel safe from getting breast cancer. There are a variety of reasons that could contribute to the lack of one type of cancer in a BRCA mutated person's family history.

- *If any men in the family have had breast cancer, that's so uncommon it's a big red flag.*
- *If there is a personal or family history of ovarian cancer, especially at a young age.*
- *If patient is of Eastern-European Jewish/ Ashkenazi ancestry. Don't automatically dismiss this. This is my link to the mutation, and I'd never even heard of the word Ashkenazi until I found out I might have the BRCA1 mutation.*
- *If patient is of French Canadian, Norwegian, Icelandic, and Dutch ancestry, she may be at increased risk.[17]*

DeAnna Howe Rice

Dear Doctors,

As a four-time BRCA breast and ovarian cancer survivor, I have a lot to say.

The most important aspect of this information for everyone who has had a member of their family diagnosed and/or dying as a result of the cancers associated with this gene, there are answers and there are ways to prevent a BRCA positive person from developing cancer. This is what we call a **Previvor**. The thought that, once identification has been made, there is a possibility of preventing the cancer from developing is exciting.

For my family, it means a possible end to much suffering.

In my case, my paternal grandmother had breast cancer in her forties and passed away at fifty-two from metastatic breast cancer to her brain. But the most obvious and glaring part of my story that should have been a red flag was my diagnosis with breast cancer at twenty-nine years of age. My doctors didn't test me!

Dr. Susan S., MD

Question for Dr. Herman

I am still not sure who to test and could you talk a bit more about insurance coverage for the testing?

Dr. Herman

Teri mentioned families with a history of pre-menopausal breast cancer, ovarian cancer diagnosed at any age, and male breast cancer should be looked at. Plus, ethnicity plays a role. HBOC is twelve and a half times more common in the Ashkenazi Jewish population. Recently added to the list of risk factors is: triple negative breast cancer — ER, PR and her2 Nu negatives.

The "Red Flags" for HBOC list includes:

- *Breast cancer before age 50*
- *Triple negative breast cancer*

- *Male breast cancer*
- *Ovarian cancer at any age*
- *Ashkenazi Jewish ethnicity*

When it comes to insurance companies: each individual insurance company has its own variation, but in general, today, most commercial insurance companies will pay for testing as long as the patient meets certain criteria. I call it "qualifying for testing." I hate when I hear a doctor say, "Insurance doesn't pay for the testing. I tell my patients it's too expensive." That's wrong.

I also hear, "How does it work with the insurance?" or "When does insurance pay for it?" In general, when the patient is at or above a five percent risk level, insurance pays. This is a good rule of thumb.

I separate the patients into two different groups:

1) *Those with cancer already*
2) *Those who don't have cancer but have a family history of breast or ovarian cancer*

Group One

Insurance is likely to pay for BRCA testing for your cancer patients if they have/had:

- *Premenopausal breast cancer*
- *Triple negative breast cancer before the age of 60*
- *Ovarian cancer at any age*

What is the insurance definition of premenopausal? It's different from the medical definition. The insurance definition of premenopausal is a woman who is fewer than fifty years old.

Fifty or more equals menopause. Statistically, if your patient is younger than fifty with breast cancer, she has about an eight percent chance of being BRCA positive. Eight percent is more than five percent. She qualifies and most insurances cover testing. Aetna[18] uses forty-five as their cut off age. So if you are over forty-five, you are menopausal. I think we would all agree that using age doesn't make the best of sense. I am sure we would rather use menopause as the criteria, but for now we use age. A red flag and qualifier would be a woman with young breast cancer even if she were the only one in her family. Test your breast cancer patients.

Next is ovarian cancer. Ovarian cancer at any age qualifies for testing. Many a healthcare professional has made the mistake of thinking, "She's diagnosed at an older age. Why would you test her?" Because ovarian cancer is age independent. The ovarian cancer patient has about a nine percent chance of being positive. Nine percent is greater than five percent, so she qualifies for testing. Test your ovarian cancer patients.

But most of my patients do not have cancer, you might say. If they have a family history how would they qualify?

Group Two

When we consider family history, for the most part, family history includes first and second-degree relatives. Father, mother, sister, brother, children are first degree. Father's father, mother's sister (aunt), mother's brother (uncle) are second-degree relatives. There must be two events in the family to qualify, a young breast cancer or ovarian cancer at any age or having been born to an Ashkenazi Jewish family (I used to call those "the big three"). But now, with triple negative (TN) breast cancer, it's the "big four" (with male breast cancer adding in a fifth element). Then there must be a second event in the family, on the same side. Either both events are on the maternal side or the paternal side. You can't have one from each. The second event can be any other breast cancer no matter the age, another ovarian cancer, bilateral breast cancer, and/or breast cancer that returned more than five years after the first diagnoses.

As a constant reminder, we should always attempt to test the family member with cancer. If the cancer patient is not tested, we might have to test all of their siblings and children. Insurance is likely to pay for BRCA testing for your patients who do not have a cancer diagnosis but have a family history if they have: At least one from each column:

A	B
☐ Breast cancer < 50 years old	☐ Breast cancer, any age
☐ TN breast cancer < than 60 years old	☐ Ovarian cancer, any age
☐ Ovarian cancer, any age	☐ Bilateral breast cancer
☐ Ashkenazi Jewish	☐ Breast cancer, five years later
☐ Male breast cancer	

Scenario One:

Your patient's mother had ovarian cancer at the age of forty-five and her grandmother had breast cancer when she was fifty-five. She also has a sister and two brothers. Each sibling has two children, a boy and a girl. Today, you are going to discuss BRCA with her. First, you would have encouraged her to have her mother tested, but you already know from her history that her mother cannot be tested, because she passed away last year.

If her mother had tested negative, the mother's siblings and children would not need testing. Now, each sibling and child will be encouraged to have it done. If your patient's test returns negative, that doesn't mean her siblings, aunts, and uncles are negative, too.

Returning to who qualifies: Your patient has a family history but no cancer. If there is no better family member available for testing, they need one of "the big four" plus another event. The other events: an additional breast cancer no matter the age, another ovarian cancer, bilateral breast cancer, breast cancer that returned more than five years after the first diagnosis.

A	B
☐ Breast cancer < 50 years old	☑ Breast cancer, any age
☐ TN breast cancer < than 60 years old	☐ Ovarian cancer, any age
☑ Ovarian cancer, any age	☐ Bilateral breast cancer
☐ Ashkenazi Jewish	☐ Breast cancer, five years later
☐ Male breast cancer	

Scenario Two:

Your patient's mother had breast cancer at the age of forty. The mother isn't available for testing. History reveals no other cancer in the family. There is only one event. "What was your mother's ethnic background?"

"Italian." Still only one event.

"Was it in one breast or both?"

"Both." Bilateral breast cancer equals two events, and your patient qualifies.

A	B
☑ Breast cancer < 50 years old	☐ Breast cancer, any age
☐ TN breast cancer < than 60 years old	☐ Ovarian cancer, any age
☐ Ovarian cancer, any age	☑ Bilateral breast cancer
☐ Ashkenazi Jewish	☐ Breast cancer, five years later
☐ Male breast cancer	

Scenario Three: (Similar story)

Your patient's mother had breast cancer at the age of forty. Her mother isn't available for testing. History reveals no other cancer in the family. There is only one event.

"What was your mother's ethnic background?"

"Italian." Still only one event.

"Was it in one breast or both?"

"Only in the right." Still only one.

"Did it ever come back?"

"Yes. She had it again when she was sixty." One person, two separate cancers, one young, a second one older; that equals two events, and she qualifies.

A	B
☑ Breast cancer < 50 years old	☐ Breast cancer, any age
☐ TN breast cancer < than 60 years old	☐ Ovarian cancer, any age
☐ Ovarian cancer, any age	☐ Bilateral breast cancer
☐ Ashkenazi Jewish	☑ Breast cancer, five years later
☐ Male breast cancer	

Scenario Four:

Your patient's mother had breast cancer at the age of sixty. History reveals no other cancer in the family. No young breast cancer. No ovarian cancer.

"What was your mother's ethnic background?"

"Ashkenazi Jewish." Ashkenazi equals one big one and breast

cancer at any age equals the second. Your patient qualifies for testing.

I've been fooled a number of times on ethnicity. I had a patient, Mrs. Rodriquez, who is Ashkenazi. People get married and change their names. Teri has noted that people may be born Jewish, but follow another religion or no religion at all and may not think to mention their Jewish heritage. Now, I don't assume. I ask.

Your patient's mother had breast cancer and there is no other cancer in the family. Questions to keep in mind:

- *At what age was she diagnosed?*
- *Was it in breast or both?*
- *Did it come back again? When?*
- *What is the ethnic background?*

A	B
☐ Breast cancer < 50 years old	☑ Breast cancer, any age
☐ TN breast cancer < than 60 years old	☐ Ovarian cancer, any age
☐ Ovarian cancer, any age	☐ Bilateral breast cancer
☑ Ashkenazi Jewish	☐ Breast cancer, five years later
☐ Male breast cancer	

Jean
You Don't Need Testing

I was treated for breast cancer in 2002. In 2005, I asked my oncologist about the BRCA test. He said to me, "You don't need that test. You've had your cancer and you're done with it."

In 2009, my gynecologist asked me if I wanted the BRCA test, and I jumped at the chance. I went back to see my oncologist and told him I was BRCA positive. I told him I was planning a PBM. I reminded him I came from Jewish heritage. He said to me, "What religion are you?" as he was fingering through my chart.

I said, "I was raised Lutheran, but my mother was Jewish."

He had a look on his face of "Boy, I blew this one."

Dr. Herman

Two additional patients you should be aware of: If there is a proven BRCA mutation in the family, that alone qualifies for testing.

When there are none of the big four — young breast cancer, triple negative breast cancer, ovarian cancer, Ashkenazi Jewish ethnicity — but there are three close relatives with breast cancer, all older than fifty, insurance will consider that as qualifying.

- *Every patient should be asked their cancer history every year (things change!)*
- *A patient with young breast cancer or ovarian cancer at any age may qualify for testing.*
- *Those without cancer usually need two events to qualify for testing.*
- *Attempts should be made to test those with cancer before testing relatives without cancer.*
- *See a list of red flags and second event scenarios above.*
- *There are always exceptions.*
- *Always utilize resources and healthcare professionals experienced in BRCA testing.*

Question from a Nurse Practitioner

I work in a very active practice. If HBOC is looking for five to ten percent of breast cancer patients, why should I spend my time looking for these patients? It seems like a lot of work for just a few people.

Dr. Herman

Your office situation seems similar to mine. In my practice, there are four physicians and a nurse practitioner. Collectively, we see four hundred to four-hundred and fifty people per week. Half of them are pregnant and half are not. Approximately twenty have a history that would qualify them for BRCA testing. Some will have already tested, few might decline testing, but the most important thing is that every patient be educated in order that they have the needed information to make informed decisions.

I will answer your question in two complementary ways. First, I will go over some numbers, and then add some perspective of what you should attempt to accomplish in your office.

Approximately 220,000 women in the United States will be diagnosed with breast cancer this year.[19] Hereditary breast and ovarian cancer syndrome is causative in five to ten percent of cases.[20]

So if we do simple math: Seven percent of 220,000 equals 15,400. Approximately 22,000 women will be diagnosed with ovarian cancer this year. Hereditary breast and ovarian cancer syndrome is causative in nine percent of cases. That is another

1,980 women. And that's just a yearly estimate.

$$15,400 + 1,980 = 17,380$$

Let's say your patient is thirty-two years old and diagnosed with breast cancer. She has tested and was found to be BRCA positive. She has a brother and a sister. On average, one will be BRCA positive. BRCA mutations are inherited autosomal dominant genes. Remember the Punnett Square from high school, big T, little t. Next, take the 15,400 breast cancer patients and add to them the 1,980 ovarian cancer patients, plus half of their siblings, half of their parents, and half of their children and you realize it is not just a few people we are talking about.

In addition, a recent study regarding low utilization of BRCA testing reported that fewer than five percent of people who should consider having BRCA testing have learned about it and followed through with testing thus far.

Fewer than five percent. We have a lot of catching up to do.

Next, some perspective:

I have been in my own office since 1993. I see approximately one-hundred women per week. That's a lot of pelvic exams and Pap smears over the years. How many ovarian cancers do you think I have found over all the years I've been in practice? Maybe one or two? Maybe? At most a few. So for all the hundreds, thousands, of pelvic exams, the yield is almost negligible. However, I keep doing pelvic exams. Why? Because for the one or two I find during the course of my career, that exam is life-changing and makes all the effort worth it. I do not believe anyone would ever suggest I should cease doing pelvic exams because I would probably find few ovarian cancers. I do not believe anyone would ever suggest I should stop looking for these patients.

I also mentioned the Pap smear. Every patient gets a Pap. In all the years in the office, I have only identified two patients with cervical cancer. Both of them are fine and well. So why should I continue doing Pap smears if my yield is so low? Because for those few I find during the course of my career, it's life-changing (indeed, possibly life-saving) for that patient and makes all the effort worth it.

Patients never tell me, "Please skip my pelvic exam. Please skip my Pap smear. Please skip my breast exam, because it is only a few people." The patients may want me to skip it. But they also want me to do everything possible to make sure that they are okay.

Katrina W.

What's my family history look like? My mom and her sister both passed from breast cancer before forty-five, their dad's sister and niece both passed of breast cancer before forty-five. All of the women on my mother's dad's side died of breast cancer before the age of forty-five. My mom's mom also died from breast cancer at the age of seventy-two.

Mother	*breast cancer <45*
Maternal aunt (mother's sister)	*breast cancer <45*
Maternal great aunt (grandfather's sister)	*breast cancer <45*
Maternal second cousin (mother's cousin)	*breast cancer <45*
Maternal grandmother	*breast cancer 70s*

As supportive as my doctor was, there was never any mention of genetic testing unless I brought it up, no mention of mammos unless I requested them. I don't understand why I have to fill out my family history if no one is doing anything with it.

I found out I was BRCA2 positive after my first appointment with Dr. Shim and Dr. Kim, part of the best breast team in the world. They listened to me, they cried with me, and they were willing to act with me. The thing is, when your family history is littered with breast cancer, you dread going to the doctor's office and filling out the family history paperwork, but if you're going to do it, guidance would be nice.

If I came to the doctor with a sore throat, a fever, white spots on my tonsils, and swollen lymph nodes, you wouldn't look at that info and walk away. You would test me for strep throat.

Every doctor would test. It's the standard of care. However, I told every doctor I saw about my family history and yet none said, "Okay, we are setting you up with a test for BRCA."

I had a bilateral prophylactic nipple-sparring mastectomy with expanders on July 10th. I had a pelvic ultrasound in June (at my request) that was clear and have had a screening in dermatology. After my breast surgeries are over, I'll have a total hysterectomy. No one had ovarian cancer but then maybe no one lived long enough for that to be a problem. I'm not taking the chance. I posted my surgery and my test results on my Facebook page.

I have a friend who has a strong family history of ovarian cancer, and she now has an appointment with her doctor to demand genetic testing, She's had no mammos, no pelvic ultrasounds, and no blood tests. She's thirty-six. Her mom died at forty-five, I think. The ball has been dropped again. I believe when you go to the doctor, you trust he or she will tell you what you need to do to live. It's just not happening at the primary care and general OB level.

My little cousin I raised who is now twenty-three was just tested: negative! How sweet is that? I have three girls: twelve, five, and two. We have a long road, but fighting isn't that bad when you know what you're fighting.

~~Dr. Veronica Sim is a breast surgeon. She is involved in developing the breast cancer high-risk clinic/prevention clinic at Oakland Kaiser. Dr. Jane H. Kim, MD a plastic surgeon has had special training in breast surgery. She practices in Oakland and Richmond, California.

- *Patients shouldn't have to request BRCA testing from you.*
- *Read patients' intake questionnaires.*
- *When the ball gets dropped as far as BRCA testing goes, this can and has resulted in DEATH. You don't want that on your conscience.*
- *Tell your patients to get tested if they should be tested.*

A Patient's Question via learnabouthboc.com:

I was diagnosed with breast cancer when I was thirty-five. Now I'm forty-five. Why hasn't my oncologist told me about BRCA during this ten-year period?

Dr. Herman

One of my great days in medicine (June 1997) was presenting

grand rounds before a group of medical oncologists. Would you believe it: a simple OB/GYN doctor giving grand rounds to oncologists? I have to go back a bit and tell you the whole story.

Two months prior, at tumor board, my patient's case was scheduled fourth in line. I patiently sat through cases number one, two, and three.

Case number two went something like this: Forty-eight-year-old female, newly diagnosed with stage IIIB ovarian cancer. Family history includes mother with breast cancer and a maternal aunt with breast cancer. At the end of the discussion, it bothered me that no one had mentioned BRCA testing as part of the treatment plan.

So from way in the back of the room, I put in my two cents. "What about BRCA testing?" All agreed it was a good idea.

Then case number three was presented: A fifty-four-year-old female, newly diagnosed with stage III ovarian cancer. Family history includes sister with breast cancer and mother with breast cancer.

Again, the case was discussed and a course of treatment was agreed upon: chemotherapy. There was no mention of BRCA testing. This time I stood up.

"Shouldn't BRCA testing be a part of the treatment plan?"

With that comment the medical oncologist leaned over to Dr. Contreras, the gynecologic oncologist, and asked, "Who is that? A geneticist?"

Dr. Contreras, in an authoritative voice, answered, "No! He's just a gynecologist who takes a history from his patients."

With that, oncology invited me to give grand rounds. I'm sure you understand. It's a good day when a gynecologist is teaching the oncologist, or so I thought it was.

All excited, I showed my PowerPoint slides, and I went through my lecture. At the end, it was time for questions and the first question threw me for a loop.

"Are you suggesting we do BRCA testing on people who don't have cancer?"

"Absolutely," I replied.

After a few more questions, my lecture had come to an end. I walked away unsure of what to think. How is it possible that the highly intelligent, highly skilled oncologist would ask me if I plan to test unaffected patients? After weeks, I finally came to a conclusion: oncologists treat cancer.

How is it that I keep seeing patients, cancer survivors, in my office who qualify for testing and have never even heard of it? Because oncologists treat cancer.

I also learned that breast surgeons operate on the breast. Oncologists treat cancer and breast surgeons operate on the breast.

For the gynecologist, the internist, the family practitioner, they spend their days doing risk-evaluation for the disease. They determine risk in order to set up risk-reducing treatment plans. It's an oversimplification, but you get the concept.

I am very happy to say that there is a noticeable transition. Recently, every oncologist, gynecologic oncologist, and breast surgeon I come across is in tune with testing high-risk family members who don't have cancer in order to avoid cancer.

Why Cancer Patients Go Untested

Here is another idea why your breast surgeon did not test you or suggest testing and why your medical oncologist did not test you or suggest testing.

All the doctors were in favor of testing. Each doctor believed that the other doctor was getting it done. The oncologist thought the breast surgeon was getting it done. The breast surgeon thought the oncologist was getting it done.

Meanwhile the oncologist was treating breast cancer and the breast surgeon was operating on the breast and as time went by it fell through the cracks.

"My oncologist wanted me to be tested, but he thought it was too much for me to handle since I was getting chemotherapy. When I was done with my treatment, I was going to go to get tested." I hear that, but we need these patients tested ASAP. BRCA testing must become a routine part of your treatment plan when the patient qualifies for testing. Keep in mind that a positive test means a change in recommendations, treatment recommendations, which can save the patient's life.

Unfortunately, there are healthcare professionals who assume that someone else has covered HBOC and BRCA mutation information. Unfortunately, there are healthcare professionals who assume it should be put off until later.

Don't be that practitioner.

Voices from the Crowd

DeAnna Howe Rice
Author, "Fight like a Mom"

To My Angel Doctor,

When I went into cardiac failure, the doctor put me on disability to see if we could stabilize my heart function and to keep it from worsening. During this time, I reflected on a very powerful interview I had done for the TV show in California, *Your Cancer Today*. I had invited a local breast surgeon, Dr. Lisa Curcio, to come on the show and speak to us about the new advances in breast cancer. I also shared that I was a two-time breast cancer survivor and still filled with so many unanswered questions. I was excited to hear everything she had to say.

She quickly stopped me. "Have you ever been tested?"

"Tested for what?" I asked almost sarcastically. I thought I had been tested for everything under the sun. This happens to be the most pivotal point in my story.

"Have you ever been tested for the BRCA gene mutation?"

"Oh, no," I explained. "They told me I had no family history."

Once again, she stopped me and looked me straight in the eyes and told me that just by virtue of my having had two breast cancers before the age of fifty, I needed to be tested. Her next question was, "Tell me anyone at all in your family who has ever had any kind of cancer, ever."

My paternal grandmother died of breast cancer. That is the only person in my entire family that had any kind of cancer. The next question, "How old was she?" I didn't know. She was my grandma, so she seemed old to me. She was sick most of my life. Double mastectomies, surgeries, she really struggled. I did some quick math and figured she died in her early fifties.

She stressed the fact that this was a test I had to have. It wasn't an option. She couldn't believe the BRCA test had never been offered, let alone encouraged. I took her seriously.

Still dealing with my heart, I made an appointment to see Dr. Curcio as a patient. She sat me down and went over all of the information regarding the details and implications of being BRCA positive or negative and how either would help to manage my care. After all, having two breast cancers before thirty-five years old is not common.

She showed me statistics and numbers; I knew why she was so insistent. I suddenly saw myself reflected in those numbers.

~~Dr. Lisa Curcio is a breast care specialist and surgeon. In August of 2005, she founded Advanced Breast Care Specialists of Orange County in Mission Viejo, CA. Dr. Curcio fought her own battle with breast cancer at age thirty-seven and has devoted her life's work to the education, prevention, and treatment of breast cancer.

Edel
I Am a BRCA-Positive Aussie

Dear Doctor, Doctors here still know hardly anything about BRCA (mutations). I have had three doctors (including one specialist) ask me what BRCA meant on my notes. I have had a couple of nurses ask me as well, and I had to explain.

What chance have we got if the doctors don't even know what BRCA means?

Amy S.

The genetic nurse said because I wasn't sure exactly where my Jewish ancestors were from, I didn't fall into the "ratio" the hospital uses to tell if testing was warranted. Also because (my sister) Kim was the only one in the family under forty when diagnosed, she said Kim's cancers (breast and ovarian) were probably a fluke. It was hard to bite my tongue at that response.

Stacey R.

This all came about because of a discussion my father had in passing with a fellow colleague. My father had somehow mentioned in the course of a conversation that many close relatives died of cancer. This colleague immediately suggested my father be tested for the broken BRCA gene. The what?

To me, what only was, just a few days ago, perhaps an encyclopedic, unknown trivia term has now come to occupy my mind most of the day. The truth is, although I can never express it, my husband and I are eternally grateful to Vicki, the in-passing colleague. It was her suggestion that my father be tested, which led me to be tested as well.

Teri's Blog
Burden of Knowledge

The genetic test itself is no more than a blood test, and it tends to take two to three weeks for the results to come back.

Some people are against the idea of being tested, even when they know the mutation runs in their family. This is obviously not the way I roll. I don't like surprises. I'm the sort of person who's been known to peek at hidden Christmas presents because I can't stand the suspense.

For me, once I knew the mutation ran in my family, I had to be tested; it wasn't even a second thought.

There is a burden of knowledge though, that much is true. I'd rather carry a burden of knowledge than an appointment card for chemo.

Dr. Herman

Teri, I love your message, *"I'd rather carry a burden of knowledge than an appointment card for chemo."* That perfectly sums it up. It resonates and I will be quoting it on and on.

Dear Practitioners,

I want you to test your patients. That is why I spent so much time working on this book. However, if I fail and not a single one of you tests one additional patient, I still consider all the effort worth it.

Why? Just take a look at the letter my fourteen-year-old daughter, Sarah, sent me from sleep-away camp last summer. I am a very proud father. You'll see; she gets it.

Sarah Herman's Postcard

"As I was texting you before, daddy, I was talking to my friend from Houston. She told me her grandmother died from breast cancer and her aunt had it twice. I told her that her family should get tested for BRCA, and I explained to her what BRCA is. I really hope she gets tested. Maybe I can go with you the next time you go to Houston, and we can make sure her family gets tested.

It might just save her life!"

Dr. Herman

A couple of years back, a fifty-four-year-old woman came to my office for a breast-check appointment.

She had felt a lump in her left breast. I took her history and learned that her mother had breast cancer and her maternal grandmother died from ovarian cancer. Those cancers didn't occur in the past five minutes. Her previous doctors never asked her the appropriate questions. Someone should have told her about BRCA mutations and had her tested years ago.

When I examined her, I knew it was breast cancer. I tested her and had her seen by the radiologist that day. Three days later, breast cancer was confirmed via pathology. She should never have been diagnosed with late-stage breast cancer. She should have never gotten cancer in the first place.

A few days later, her BRCA test came back positive for a mutation. Even worse, she told me she couldn't tell anyone about it. She had breast cancer. She was BRCA positive and it had to remain a secret, because her daughter was getting married the next week.

I hate these types of stories, and there are a lot of them out there. Below are some ideas, concepts and views that I hope will help you with your patients.

Comment from A New Jersey Physician

Dr. Herman, I appreciate that you test and care for many BRCA-positive patients and their families. You are obviously passionate about what you do. However, I cannot do the same, because my patient population is fundamentally different from yours. Your patients want testing while mine do not.

Dr. Herman
Testing

I have thought about my response to this question as I see and hear stories of patients going untested. I believe that my patients are exactly like yours. I know they are. I one-hundred-percent agree that most do not want to be tested. Your patients don't want to be tested and neither do mine.

Concepts from Grand Rounds

I have given over five-hundred BRCA-related talks. It's a dynamic process, and I'm always redoing my slides. They keep changing as new information is reported. There are, however, ideas, themes I always try to get across.

BRCA testing falls under the risk evaluation and risk-reduction model. In regard to tests I offer in my office, my patients don't want to be tested for most of them.

When lecturing, I often ask rhetorically, *What do I do as an OB/GYN?* I deliver babies, of course. When not on labor and delivery or operating, most often you will find me in the office seeing patients. In the office, I am focused on evaluating my patient's risk for cervical cancer, endometrial cancer, breast cancer, and prenatal care such as Down Syndrome education and assessment. In other words, I spend my days evaluating risk: risk evaluation. Then I create a plan for risk reduction.

Risk evaluation and risk reduction. That's how I think of BRCA testing. You should, too.

There are many parallels between BRCA testing and other testing in the office. When lecturing, I always begin with the most common procedure I do in the office: The dreaded Pap smear.

Every OB/GYN I have ever met, without exception, agrees

that many of their patients don't know why they are even having a Pap smear. When lecturing in Dallas, Texas, they taught me why women have Pap smears: It's so they can get their birth control pills. Good point! Some women tell me that the Pap is a test used to detect cancer, ovarian cancer, uterine cancer. Others have no idea at all.

Cancer.gov defines a Pap as "*a procedure in which cells are scraped from the cervix for examination under a microscope. It is used to detect cancer and changes that may lead to cancer. A Papanicolaou test can also show conditions, such as infection or inflammation that are not cancer.*"[21]

In other words, it's a risk evaluation tool. Even if the patient understands what the Pap is used for, in all likelihood, she couldn't interpret the results. She can't tell you what HGSIL, LGSIL and ASCUS are. And, last I heard, it's not a lot of fun to have a Pap smear. These are realities. The patient doesn't know why she is having a Pap, she can't interpret her cytology report, and the test is not fun to have. Meanwhile, she still does it. Why? Because she relies on me to do what I need to do to take care of her. I need to figure out her risk of cervical cancer in order to reduce that risk: risk evaluation then risk reduction.

Let's look at another test. The next test I commonly perform is called a Pipelle®. A forty-seven-year-old woman came to my office complaining of abnormal vaginal bleeding. She needed the bleeding to stop.

So I say, "I can stop your bleeding, but before I do that, I need to get a sample. I need to do a Pipelle®."

Why didn't I say an endometrial biopsy? Because, it might add to her worry. No need for that. Then I explain, "I'm going to make sure this bleeding is nothing important. I'm going to make sure that there isn't anything significant going on. I need to evaluate your risk. We're going to move to the exam room. It causes some cramps. Most women do just fine."

What happens? She has the Pipelle® and it does cause some cramps, sometimes bad, sometimes not so bad. She waits a week, more or less, and the pathology report comes in. She can't interpret that report.

She doesn't know what hyperplasia is, hyperplasia with atypia or hyperplasia without atypia. She can't interpret the results but she still went ahead and got tested. Why? Because she relies on me, her healthcare professional, to do what I needed to do in order take care of her. I need to figure out what the risk is in order to go ahead and reduce that risk. It is a risk evaluation tool for me so I can better take care of my patient.

Mindful of the above, we turn to BRCA testing. In my view, BRCA testing has many parallel components. It is a risk evaluation tool. The information allows the healthcare professional to more accurately evaluate risk and then render better care: risk evaluation and risk reduction.

I have met with doctors all over the country who agree with the doctor from New Jersey. They tell me that they don't do BRCA tests because their patients aren't interested.
Patients are interested.

As a general rule, if it's important for the healthcare professional, then it becomes important for the patient. The test needs to be explained, the who, what, where, when, and why. With explanation, in most cases, your patients will test. Go ahead and explain why the test is important and that the testing is available in order to render better care. In other words, counseling. She will respond to counseling and will do what needs to be done. When counseled, an educated patient can and will make informed choices about BRCA testing.

Here are some take home concepts:

- *We do risk evaluations and risk reductions.*
- *Patients don't desire to be tested for anything, in general.*
- *Patients test because you tell them it's important for their care.*
- *BRCA testing is risk evaluation tool.*
- *BRCA testing may lead to risk reduction of breast and ovarian cancer.*
- *Proper education (also known as counseling) equals BRCA testing.*

DeAnna Howe Rice
They Tell Me

Dear Doctors, Please, please, practice good medicine. And educate your patients not only about HBOC, but genetic testing. Then sleep soundly at night knowing that you have done your job and hopefully, saved lives, too.

I lecture all over the US about BRCA. I am a patient and a lecturer. I think I may have heard it all as I travel the country lecturing and speaking with healthcare professionals.

Below is what I call the list of excuses:

They tell me, "My patients don't want to know."

They tell me, "My patients can't afford the test, so I'm not even going to tell them about it."

They tell me, "My patients don't have insurance, so I'm not going to tell them about it."

They tell me, "I don't have patients like that."

They tell me, "It's not my job."

They tell me they'll test to appease me; they lie.

They tell me, "I don't have extra time to talk to my patients."

They tell me, "Breast cancer can only come from the mother's side."

They tell me, "I just don't have enough information."

They tell me, "I don't know what to do once they receive their result."

They tell me, "I can't see the benefits of testing."

They tell me, "I am already taking care of the patients. They get mammograms."

They tell me, "I worry that my patients may become depressed."

They tell me that the patients may be discriminated against. Worst of all of these excuses is, "I can't make money discussing testing. It will cost me to counsel these patients."

Every one of these excuses is nonsense and heinous. These are human lives we are talking about: someone's mother, daughter, sister, wife, best friend, aunt, or cousin.

A doctor's job is to inform and provide excellent medical care for us. If there is a test that can save lives, I believe it is their responsibility to inform us and stress the importance of the test. Do not make excuses. Get testing.

Dr. Herman
Low Risk, High Risk, Extreme Risk

Overall, a woman's chance of getting breast cancer during her life is one in eight, or about twelve percent.[22] That's considered low risk. If a woman's mother had breast cancer, the risk jumps to about twenty percent. That's called high risk. If a woman has a BRCA mutation, the risk goes up over the fifty percent range, and in some instances higher than seventy percent. Some would call that extreme risk. I certainly would.

I think of BRCA as a test I use to help define my patient's risk. What category does she fall into: low, high, or extreme? I also utilize other tests to help define risk: personal history, family history, breast exams, mammography, and breast ultrasound. BRCA is a risk evaluation tool that helps me help the patient.

I like to ask at risk patients, "What's your risk for breast cancer?"

They look at me and say, "You should know. You're the doctor." I have a test that helps me figure it out: the BRCA test.

- *By age 50, 2% of women in the general population and 33-50% of BRCA mutation positive women will be diagnosed with breast cancer*
- *By age 70, 7% of women in the general population and 56-87% of BRCA mutation positive women will be diagnosed*

with breast cancer

- *By age 70, 1.2% of women in the general population and 27-44% of BRCA mutation positive women will be diagnosed with ovarian cancer[23]*

Important Points:

- *Family histories are going unrecognized.*
- *Women are getting cancer because their histories are going unrecognized.*
- *Dr. H's fourteen-year-old daughter, Sarah, is identifying possible BRCA families.*
- *Your patients don't want Pap smears, endo-biopsies, mammos, or BRCA testing.*
- *Your patients would rather get tested than go for chemo.*
- *Your patients would rather not have any testing if they didn't have to.*
- *BRCA testing is a risk evaluation tool.*
- *Your patients get better treatment plans when you have more accurate information.*
- *If BRCA testing is important to you, then it will be important to your patients.*
- *There are many excuses providers use for why they don't test their patients.*
- *What is your patient's risk for breast cancer: low, high, or extreme?*
- *Many times, patients have preconceived misconceptions about BRCA testing.*

Voices from the Crowd

Karen
Israel, From BRACHA.org

I have been living in Israel for the past twenty years but was born and raised in London. I have always been proactive about my health, because from a very young age, my family has been blighted with breast and ovarian cancer.

When I was fourteen years old, and my aunt was forty, she complained of a simple bloated stomach. After being told a number of times by her doctor not to worry, she was sent to do some more extensive tests, which took several weeks. She was finally diagnosed with ovarian cancer, by which time, the disease had progressed extensively throughout her ovaries and womb.

She underwent chemotherapy treatment, which in those days involved a three-day stay in hospital during each treatment. Sadly, she died nine months later.

In 1990, at age forty-six, my mother was diagnosed with breast cancer. My mother had a lumpectomy, chemotherapy, and radiation. However, three years later, the cancer returned to her lungs and then a few months afterward, to her liver. Sadly, she died in 1994, aged fifty. Although my aunt had died of ovarian cancer and my mother of breast cancer, we did not see any link between the two and thought of it as no more than just a tragic coincidence that two sisters were diagnosed with cancer at a relatively young age.

In the early 2000s, I read reports that suggest some breast cancers and ovarian cancers are caused by a series of genetic mutations. This is when it first occurred to me that there may be a link between my aunt's ovarian cancer and my mother's breast cancer. I enquired at my local genetics clinic about pursuing genetic testing. I had already decided that if I tested positive for a BRCA1 or BRCA2 mutation I would have a prophylactic double mastectomy and an oophorectomy. Fortunately, I did not have to go down that route, because the test result came out negative.

My two younger sisters were not interested in pursuing genetic testing. This was on the basis that even if they had opted to do the test, and if the test came out positive, they would not consider having mastectomy and/or an oophorectomy. They believed it would be pointless doing the test in the first place. They both were young and single and viewed these surgical options as drastic self-mutilation. In addition, they felt that the operation would make them lose their femininity, and that they would inevitably find it hard to meet potential partners.

This bad decision was to change our entire lives at the end of 2002. My youngest sister, Sharron, was diagnosed with breast cancer at age twenty-nine. We were all shocked and horrified. She was so young, over fifteen years younger than our aunt and mother were at diagnosis! Sharron was in the prime of her life, living a fast-paced lifestyle working in IT recruitment during the week and teaching and performing salsa dancing on weekends and evenings.

She discovered a lump whilst in Europe on holiday with her boyfriend of two years. Sharron was told by the doctors that she had a ninety-six percent chance of making the five-year mark, after which one is considered to be in remission. It was at this point that Sharron decided to proceed with genetic testing and discovered that she was a carrier of the BRCA2 genetic mutation.

Sharron proceeded with treatment, and then continued where she left off living a fast-paced lifestyle, working hard and dancing in her spare time. Two years later, she discovered her cancer had returned to her bones, gradually spreading throughout the rest of her body over the next three years before she tragically died in September 2007, aged thirty-four. The positive result enabled our other sister and our cousins to make the choice of whether to have the genetic test or not.

If my sister, Sharron, had only considered having the genetic test prior to her diagnosis, and had opted to have prophylactic double mastectomy and oophorectomy, then who knows? Perhaps she would still be around today to tell her own story.

Karen's Story In-Review

- *Maternal aunt, ovarian cancer at age 40, dies at 41*
- *Mother, breast cancer at age 46, dies at 50*
- *Karen tests negative*
- *Sisters don't test (lack of knowledge)*
- *Youngest sister, Sharron, breast cancer at 29*
- *Can't believe how young breast cancer appeared*
- *Sharron tests BRCA positive*
- *Sharron passes away at 34*
- *Family history doesn't determine how young BRCA breast cancer can strike*
- *Sharron might still be alive if she had tested at the outset*

Risk Assessment for Hereditary Cancer Syndromes[24]

Name_____Date_____

*Instructions: Please circle Y to those that apply to YOU and/or YOUR FAMILY (on both your **mother's** & **father's** side).Beside each statement, please list relationship to you (self, paternal uncle, maternal aunt, paternal grandmother) and their age at diagnosis.*

BREAST AND OVARIAN CANCER		RELATIONSHIP	AGE
Y / N	Breast cancer at age 50 or younger	1)	
		2)	
		3)	
		4)	
Y / N	Breast cancer older than 50	1)	
		2)	
		3)	
		4)	
Y / N	Breast cancer in both breasts or cancer that came back more than 5 years after diagnosis	1)	
		2)	
Y / N	Ovarian cancer at any age	1)	
		2)	
Y / N	Both breast and ovarian cancer in any one person	1)	
		2)	
Y / N	Ashkenazi Jewish ancestry (European Jews)		

Dr. Herman

Physicians and patients have additional concerns about testing: Many physicians tell me that they don't have their patients tested because it's not covered by insurance.

Wrong answer!

Testing is covered by insurance and it has been for a long time now. Almost every commercial/private insurance covers testing for those that have a significant personal and/or history of cancer in their family. If the patient doesn't have insurance or their plan doesn't cover it, as providers it is our job to encourage the patient to test as indicated medically and the patient must then decide what to do.

Many physicians are still reluctant.

If a physician sends a patient for a mammogram and the radiologist sends a report saying an MRI of the breast is indicated, you call the patient and send her for that MRI. If her insurance will not approve it, you document in the chart that you told the patient to go. The patient then decides if she will spend the money. An MRI of the breast is $1,000 to $3,000. It is not your job to say, "You don't need to do the MRI because your insurance will not pay for it."

Marilyn

Dear Dr. D.A., I have a strong family history for both breast and ovarian cancer. Two months ago, I finally tested and tested positive for BRCA2. Two years ago, when I discussed testing with you, you dissuaded me from testing because the test cost a lot. Now I find out from your partner that my insurance covers it and has covered it for many years. Even if it weren't covered, I would have done it anyway. In the future, please give us the proper information and we will make (our own) choices.

Ellin W.

Dear Dr. Herman,

I was at a bridal shower yesterday, and I met a mother and two daughters who are appropriate candidates for testing. The daughter, who lives in Queens, New York, will be calling you for an appointment. I only had your cell and home number, so I gave her your cell. Hope that's okay.

For your information, her sister, who is in her thirties, was told, "Absolutely do not test, because, once your insurance gets hold of results, you are done."

That sister lives in New Jersey, where not only do we have GINA and HIPPA but the best laws in the nation for health, life, short- and long-term care, and disability. As you know, there has never been a case upheld for discrimination.

I tried to explain that it's their history that gets them. Test results will tell you that you are not as high risk as could be, or that you are, and you can change medical management to decrease risk.

The mother wants the daughters to test (was not aware of paternal link); the New Jersey sister seems tougher to test. The Queens sister seems more willing to understand the benefit.

Dr. Herman
On the Gina Law

Thanks, Ellen. I agree with you. I've had similar experiences. Many physicians tell me that they don't have their patients tested because their patient might lose their insurance coverage if they are positive. Wrong! Testing will not cause your patients to lose her insurance.

From the inception of testing in 1994, both practitioner and patient have worried about health insurance discrimination but over the years I don't think it ever happened. I searched for and could not identify a single report. Almost two decades later, the facts on the ground say there is no real threat of discrimination.

In 1998, a national law was written that makes it illegal to discriminate based on genetic testing results. The Genetics Information Nondisclosure Act, GINA, was signed into law by the then President Bush in on May 21, 2008.

Teri's Blog
What Does GINA Say?

So what does the GINA law say? Basically this law makes it illegal for health insurance companies or employers to discriminate against people with faulty DNA. What that means is that insurance companies aren't allowed to deny coverage or charge higher rates because of a genetic mutation that increases the risk of certain diseases. It also states that employers can't base decisions of hiring, firing, or promotion based on genetic predispositions either.

Dr. Herman
Insurance Agent's View of Genetic Discrimination

I once discussed the entire discrimination issue with an insurance agent, and he told me patients with a family history who test negative for BRCA may be entitled to a reduction in premium. Because of the family history, they are being charged more, and now they have a valid claim that it doesn't run in the family and they shouldn't be penalized. I get that.

Discrimination should no longer be and should never have been an obstacle to testing. If your patient is at risk for hereditary breast and ovarian cancer syndrome get them tested.

Question from Teri's Blog

I have a friend whose mother had cancer, and so did her mother, and her mother, etc… not to mention several aunts. How do you convince a friend to go get tested (when you wouldn't think you need to)? I am just not as well informed about any of this stuff and don't want to sound stupid.

Dr. Herman's Response

You shouldn't have to convince her to test. You have to convince her to get educated. Tell her that she needs to be properly educated before deciding to be tested or not. Have the names and numbers of the best genetic counselors and practitioners ready for her.

Question from an OB/GYN

I have a thirty-five-year-old patient who should be tested. She declined. I think she may be a BRCA mutation carrier. How do I manage her?

Dr. Herman
Misconceptions

It is very hard to manage these patients. It goes back to the low risk, high risk, extreme risk. Which category does she fall into? Sounds like high or extreme. So either you have to guess or you have to get the information.

It is always the patient's right not to test. I do, however, believe that if she has the necessary information to make an informed decision, she will choose to be tested. I have talked with many healthcare professionals on the topic of how to speak with patients who decline testing because they "don't want to know."

Below I've included some thoughts and suggestions:

As a practitioner, one of the first things I do is make sure my patient is aware I know the entire subject of hereditary cancer is not an easy topic to think about or talk about. I explain that we must have an educated discussion because this is necessary to make an informed decision. She must have a solid explanation of why her history is significant for hereditary cancer testing and how a positive result, as well as negative result, will help in management and the repercussions for the family. I am constantly reminding patients of the goal to keep them healthy.

I inquire as to why she does not want to know. Often, the answer is based on misconception. When that misconception is corrected, she can make a proper informed decision.

One of the most common misconceptions that I hear is, "I don't want to test because I will have to have a mastectomy if my test comes back positive." By far that's number one.

I like to ask, "If you didn't have to have a mastectomy, would you test?"

The answer comes back, "Yeah, I would test."

"Well, you don't have to have a mastectomy. It's just one of the options. Now, let me give you the information you need."

Two more of the common misconceptions are: threat of discrimination and the cost of genetic testing. We've touched on both of those above. Compared to the way it was even two years ago, many more patients are informed about the GINA law and the protections it affords against discrimination based on genetic testing. As far as insurance coverage goes, most insurance companies pay for those who qualify for testing.

Another misconception I hear from time to time is that a positive test result means cancer now or guaranteed cancer in the future. It is time to reassure your patient this is just not the case. This is a good opportunity to reassure her that there are well-defined management options to help avoid getting cancer. I remind my patients that BRCA testing is a risk evaluation tool that helps me take care of them better. Once I am able to evaluate risk effectively, I am able to reduce the risk equal to or even less than the general population. Numerous studies have proven clinical utility and cost effectiveness of BRCA testing.

There are other patients who decline testing because they are not ready to undergo any surgery. They agree that, when ready, they will test. They think they are obligated have surgery if they are BRCA positive. They are unaware that many of my patients have chosen options other than surgery such as surveillance and chemoprevention. Surveillance and/or chemoprevention are proven options for the breasts. These patients need to be properly informed that surgery is one of the options, not the only one.

When speaking about ovaries and tubes, the timing of surgery and the procedure for removing adnexa is imperative (after thirty-five and when done childbearing).

Treatment Options for Patients with Positive Test Results

Increased Surveillance, Chemoprevention, Risk-Reducing Surgery

I believe one of the most important factors in your patient's decision to test or not is her understanding of how the information helps the healthcare professional. I can't stress this enough.

Consider the difference between these two statements:

I would like you to think about testing…

~Versus~

I need the information from this test…

When your patient understands the difference between:

I can manage you based on less accurate information…

~Versus~

I can manage you based on more accurate information from this test…

…she will recognize the value of testing.

A patient should never feel pressured into testing. If she needs time to review, to think it over, to do more research, to formulate questions, she should always be allowed and encouraged to do this. However, as practitioners, we realize we must ensure we have a good follow-up system in place. It would be a good idea to have her set up a follow-up visit before she leaves your office.

After testing, when I speak with patients and inquire as to the deciding factor for testing, I find that what really convinced them to test were their children. General rule: people often do things for their children that they wouldn't normally consider for themselves.

Here is a really important point: If your patient declines testing this year, it doesn't mean she will decline testing later on. Don't be afraid to revisit or bring up the issue again and discuss it. I tell my patients that, not only will I bring it up every year, I will also let them know what is new in the BRCA world. It is amazing to me what we have learned in the last decade. I am excited about the new information that will be available in a decade to come.

Question from a Nurse Practitioner

I identify all the patients who should have BRCA testing. I send them to the genetic counselor. A year later I find out that they never made it there. What am I supposed to do?

Dr. Herman

It is sad to think that a woman might end up with cancer because she never made it to the genetic counselor. I hope that doesn't happen to your patients. It seems to me that is a much more common event than many will admit. Some estimates say sixty to seventy percent never go.

There are numerous barriers to overcome in order to get the patient there.

Genetic Counselor

I am a genetic counselor. I spend a lot of time with the patients when they come in. When finished with the counseling session, the patients are asked to go home and make an appointment for testing if they decide to test. A lot of the patients don't return. What are your thoughts?

Dr. Herman

I have been faced with this question many times. I started out this way as well: "Go home and think about it," but realized very quickly that patients were not returning. I would identify with my patient, discuss the options, and counsel her. She seemed very interested in testing. I would give her a brochure, and I would wait a week and another week. A month would go by and nothing.

As above, you need this information in order to extend the best care to your patients. If you don't express that these test results are important to you then certainly your patients assume it's not. You need to let them know the importance.

A scenario: A patient comes to my office. She is forty-three

years old and has three children. I go over her history. She has
no breast or ovarian cancer in her family. I am still concerned
about her breast health. I let her know there is a test I could
send her for. I explain there is a breast center where she could
go and at that center, professionals will check her breasts.

"They will start by squeezing your breasts between two metal
plates. After your breasts are sufficiently squished, they will
shoot radiation at them." Just then, I hand her a brochure and
tell her, "If you want this done, let me know and I will set it all
up. If you do not want to do it, then that is okay, too."

I will bet you she will never end up having a mammography if
that's the way it's presented.

I like this next example, too. The last patient's sister comes to
the office a week later. She is twenty-eight years old and is in
very good health. As part of her yearly checkup I explain to
her that I'm going to take this metal clamp thing and I'm going to put it in her vagina. Often the metal clamp thing is cold.
It is not very comfortable and most women don't like it. Then,
I give her a brochure and tell her to read it and let me know if
she desires this test. I will bet you that she, as well as most of
my other patients, would never end up having a Pap smear.

The bottom line is if the information is important to you as a
practitioner you should let your patient know it. If she knows
it is important to you, she will usually follow through and
have the testing done.

- *With a significant history, insurance pays for BRCA testing.*
- *Cost is not a reason not to tell your patients about BRCA.*
- *The GINA law protects your patients from insurance and
  employment discrimination.*
- *Your patients may believe surgery is the only plan when*

BRCA *positive*.

- *If you send a patient for genetic counseling, make sure they go (in other words: follow up with them).*
- *Your patients will test if you express that you need this information in order to take care of them.*
- *If your patient declines testing now, don't be afraid to revisit testing at the next appointment.*
- *If testing isn't important to you, it will not be important to your patient.*

Voices from the Crowd

Rebecca W.
Peace of Mind

Being tested has given me some peace of mind, and I feel in control of my future.

Raechel Maki
My Mother

My mother died after a four-year difficult battle with ovarian cancer. Five months of remission out of four years. She never gave up trying to beat her cancer, even after the doctors told her to go home and enjoy the last few months she had left to live. If she would have had the opportunity to know prior to her diagnosis that she was genetically predisposed to breast/ovarian cancer she would have done anything and everything she could have to live.

Teri's Blog
I'm Angry

Doctors need to BRCA test their patients and break the cycle of cancer in these families.

- *I'm angry that I know people who have lost their loved ones at far too young an age to these genetic cancers.*
- *I'm angry that I see my friends having their hearts ripped out as they find out they or their sisters, mothers, aunts, daughters, and fathers have cancer that they may not live through.*
- *I'm angry that my aunt died of ovarian cancer.*
- *I'm angry that my own mother is in the final stage of it.*
- *I'm angry that I can't do more to help.*

Amy S.
Plenty of Time

Frustration. I'm still in my twenties. I hear a lot, that I have plenty of time left before I have to worry about such things. I look at my sister who was in her early thirties when she was diagnosed with breast cancer and is now dying of both breast and ovarian cancer in her late thirties, all because people didn't allow her the chance that I have been given. I'd be a fool to play with those odds.

Teri's Blog
Holy Hell and Woe is Me

I can either look at this BRCA mutation as: holy hell, woe is me. O-M-G, the sky is falling, or I can look at it as a blessing. Believe me, there are days when I feel sorry for myself, when I can't believe that, as a gift to myself for my thirty-ninth birthday, I had my reproductive organs removed.

Mostly, I try to focus on the good things that are coming from it. Number one, I don't have to die from breast or ovarian cancer. I was lucky enough to learn of my mutation and have the choice to do something about it before anything bad happened. I beat ovarian cancer before it ever had a chance to get me! I beat breast cancer, too. I'm not a survivor. I am a Previvor.

That was a good birthday present. So many others have not been so lucky.

Raechel Maki
I Cannot Pass up the Chance

I have been given an opportunity my mother never would have passed up, and out of respect for her and all other women who have fought courageous battles against these horrible diseases, I cannot pass up the chance to be a Previvor. Cancer Previvor is the only kind of cancer patient I ever want to be described as.

Stephanie Bangal
Don't Wait

The advice I would give someone is simple: take care of yourself and don't wait to find out about something that could have been prevented earlier. Don't miss an opportunity.

Jackie M.
How You Should Treat Us

In explaining things, treat us like intelligent people (my own gynecologic oncologist does this very well, but I've had doctors treat me in a patronizing manner). Although most of us are not super familiar with the background literature, we recognize that we have the capacity to understand what all of this means if explained well. Try and gauge what our current level of knowledge is and go from there. I think the really big thing here is to really listen to our questions and concerns.

Jenny D.
Touch and Inspire

I don't know if my story may touch or inspire you, but I do know that with all of my heart, I have extended my own life by being pro-active and making hard choices and removing the parts of me that could potentially change my story from something "positive."

Treatment Options

Teri's Blog
November 2009

Since I learned of my BRCA1 positive status (February 2009), I've thought of so many things. Should I have a hysterectomy and an oophorectomy? Or just the oophorectomy and skip the hysterectomy? What about instant menopause or hormone replacement therapy? Should I have my breasts removed? Which reconstruction option should I choose, if any? Which doctor should I go to?

I had months and months to learn about my health. I've had time to research doctors and all things BRCA. I'm lucky because I have the chance to be proactive instead of being put in a position of being reactive.

Of course I have the fear that the cancer may be silently growing right now as I type this but the better chance is that I will get those trouble parts out of my body before the cancer can attack. I've had time to come to terms with my decisions.

Dr. Herman
Background Information

These are the main treatment options including surveillance; chemoprevention; and risk-reducing surgery, mastectomy and

BSO. I happen to use the terminology "risk-reducing" in place of the word prophylactic because both patients and providers understand what risk-reducing surgery means.

Surveillance for breast cancer includes breast exams, mammography, and breast MRI with contrast from around twenty-five-years old. Surveillance doesn't decrease the chance of getting breast cancer. It allows for earlier detection and with that comes better outcomes. As for ovarian cancer surveillance, it has been suggested that a routine of pelvic ultrasound and CA-125 every six months can be employed. I have found no support for this in the literature, nor have I ever had a single OB/GYN who is willing to tell me he/she believes in ovarian cancer surveillance for their own family members or their patients.

Chemoprevention for breast cancer prevention may include Tamoxifen[25] and potentially Raloxifene[26]. They are thought to decrease recurrent ER+breast cancer in the general breast cancer population by fifty and thirty-three percent, respectively. This seems to hold true in preventing breast cancer in the non-affected BRCA patient. Studies are ongoing. But what about ovarian cancer risk reduction? It appears that oral contraceptives (OCPs), the only known medication that decreases the risk of ovarian cancer, does so in BRCA patients as well.

I inform my patients that risk-reducing surgery reduces the risks by ninety-five to ninety-seven percent. That's mastectomy for breast and BSO for ovarian. There's a bonus for those having a BSO before menopause: not only is the risk of ovarian cancer reduced but BSO also reduces the risk of breast cancer by approximately fifty percent.

Risk-Reducing Measures

- *Tamoxifen reduces risk of breast cancer 5%*
- *Mastectomy reduces breast cancer risk 90%*
- *Oophorectomy reduces ovarian cancer risk 96%*
- *Oophorectomy reduces breast cancer risk up to 68%*
- *Oral Contraceptives reduce risk of ovarian cancer up to 60%*

Teri
Reducing my Risk

I always knew this on some level, but after all I've been through, I truly realize that breasts and ovaries don't make a woman.

Being strong enough, and selfless enough to cut our lifetime risk of breast cancer from eighty-seven percent down to less than two percent, and ovarian cancer from forty-four percent down to less than two percent, swallowing our sense of vanity and what makes us feel pretty, to avoid a lifetime of worry, wondering when that big ticking C-bomb is going to drop, loving ourselves and our families enough to go through the emotional and physical pain of willingly losing parts of our body, to live mostly free of fear, that is what makes a woman beautiful.

Teri's Blog, 2009
The Day before My MRI

I've never had a breast MRI before, or even a mammogram. Funny words for me to say, since I also have an appointment to have a double mastectomy soon! Speaking of funny, I have a group of friends who also have BRCA mutations, and I was asking them what I should expect of the breast MRI. When it was described to me, my jaw sort of dropped. It sounds a little embarrassing, truth be told. I have a curious mind, so of course, I had to do a Google image search to see what it looks like. Try it; you'll see what I mean!

Oh, and some of the girls had vitamin E or other such things taped/glued to their nipples for the procedure.

Yeah, it seems I'm in for a real treat. Oh, the indignity of it all! Well, as my grandpa always used to say, "What are ya gonna do?" Exactly, nothing, I'm just going to go with it.

Gretchen O.
On Tamoxifen

Hello all, I wanted to share my experience with taking Tamoxifen with you. I may eventually have a PBM but I wanted to take some time deciding and wanted to reduce my risk right away. I chose to take Tamoxifen. I think the Tamoxifen option is not offered very much, even though it could really work for certain women.

I am premenopausal and have never had cancer. I'm very healthy. The only side effects I have experienced are slightly drier skin and a longer menstrual cycle (twenty-nine instead of twenty-six days). I think I actually might sleep better on the stuff. The many doctors I have spoken with tell me women with my health profile have similar experiences to mine on Tamoxifen.

Bottom line: It doesn't cause menopause in healthy premenopausal women who have not had cancer, as many women seem to believe. And it is a breast cancer risk-reduction option for BRCA positive women. Also, the chances of having a thrombic event, uterine sarcoma, or endometrial cancer in healthy, premenopausal women below age fifty on Tamoxifen are very, very low.

Teri
Tamoxifen

Thanks, Gretchen. I believe the concern most of us have with taking Tamoxifen as a chemoprevention drug is that it has shown to potentially cause uterine cancer. To me, it seemed like trading one bad risk for another bad risk.

Patricia D. (New York)
Mammography / MRI vs. Mastectomy

I have a family history of breast cancer, ovarian cancer, and colon cancer. At fifty-two years old, I learned I am also positive for the BRCA1 mutation. I was advised to have surgery to remove my ovaries and fallopian tubes. There was no doubt in my mind this was the right thing to do. Surgery was scheduled and thankfully there was no cancer.

I was also advised of the various options for my breasts, including surveillance, medication and/or surgery. I could continue surveillance, and that is what I chose to do. I knew I must be diligent in going for testing every six months. First, an MRI was scheduled. I am extremely claustrophobic; an MRI is not an easy test for me. Here is my first tip: With enough Valium, even I can have an MRI. So I did.

Now my screenings would include annual MRIs, a sonogram every six months, along with a mammogram annually. The alternative to all of this is a mastectomy with reconstruction.

Even though I had a breast biopsy in October 2007, I decided to continue testing and early detection was fine for me.

Before I knew it, four months had passed since my MRI and it was time to schedule a mammogram and sonogram and then a MRI and then a sono and then a mammo. Time goes so fast!

Suddenly, I always had the tests in the back of my mind. I found myself stressed about what would show up this time? Would I need another biopsy?

I remember and relive what occurred when I had the biopsy. The time from scheduling the biopsy to the actual procedure and waiting for the results was a nightmare. Fortunately, those results were benign. I was so certain about my decision to continue testing every six months and now I was suddenly questioning my decision and found myself very confused.

I spoke to my doctors and people who have experienced similar situations. After much consideration, I have accepted the fact that diligent surveillance is not working for me.

Debra
BRACHA.ORG.IL

I am an American currently living in Israel. My story starts with my father. He had his first cancer at age fifty-seven, a malignant melanoma. At age seventy-four, he got breast cancer. I couldn't believe it. My vigorous and strong father getting all these terrible cancers. Not one of his doctors recommended he get tested for any hereditary syndrome.

I was curious, so I Googled all his cancers and especially typed in "male breast cancer." The Google results showed he could have the BRCA mutation.

I realized the likelihood of him carrying a genetic mutation was very high. He agreed to be tested only for the sake of my sister and myself. He never wanted to know what his status was. He turned out to be BRCA2 positive (6174DelT), one of the common Jewish mutations.

I now had something to explain why he was prone to getting these cancers. I knew from my research I had a fifty percent chance of inheriting the mutation. I decided to arm myself with all the information that I could gather and made an appointment for my own genetic counseling.

Unfortunately, a few days before my visit, my beloved father lost his fight for life at age seventy-seven. I had to cancel my appointment and finally rescheduled it two months later. My father and I shared many things, like the dark circles around our eyes and our love of sports. I felt we were always connected in many ways.

When it came back positive, I was not too shocked.

I knew that I was the type of person who could not live with the day-to-day worry of, "am I going to get cancer today?" I was already age fifty-one and I felt like my breasts were like "ticking time bombs." I knew I wanted a prophylactic mastectomy right away. I was already in natural menopause and knew I also wanted a prophylactic hysterectomy and an oophorectomy.

Amy Shainman
Doing Nothing or Doing Something

For me, I saw only two choices in front of me: do nothing or do something. I could sit around with my high-risk percentages and dense breasts and wait to see if I would get cancer or I could have prophylactic surgeries and virtually cure myself before any issue of cancer would arise. I watched what my sister, Jan, and my friend, Kristin, were going through. **Cancer.**

I thought, *Yes, I have inherited this very dangerous genetic mutation, but I have been given the gift of having options to drastically reduce my cancer risk. Knowing I can actually do something to prevent what they are going through and even avoid death. I can't just sit on this knowledge and do nothing.*

Teri
Self-Empowered

Having learned as much as I could about it, I have taken charge of my own life. I've empowered myself. I decided to give the finger to my pre-disposition to cancer. Yeah, the middle one. Right now, thinking about it, it feels good. Yes, I knew the recovery was going to be rough, but having met many, many women who've gone through this before me, and lived through it, gives me strength. Knowing so many who are done, healed, and at the end of their journey, they are happy and that gives me hope.

Doesn't Doubt Decision

A fellow blogger, Kayleigh, is dealing with breast cancer. She's about to go through a very aggressive round of chemo. I feel sick for her; I wish she didn't have to deal with this. I wish she had known before the cancer struck, so that she could be in my situation of fighting the cancer before it even appears. I feel lucky for knowing about my BRCA1 mutation beforehand, but I still think it sucks that I have it, and it sucks that so many of us have to go through this.

Sue Friedman, Founder of FORCE: Facing Our Risk of Cancer Empowered

Sue said it best when she said, "It is wonderful to be grateful to be alive but it shouldn't be a requirement placed on us by others. It is okay to want it all."

Voices from the Crowd

Gail Mankiewicz
Tamoxifen

I was offered Tamoxifen and/or Raloxifen, because I was just going into menopause at the time, and I was fairly healthy (but had cysts on ovaries and surgery revealed more on the fallopian tubes and fibroid tumors in my uterus, plus an abnormal Pap).

I just kept thinking, *This is a form of chemotherapy, and I just don't want to go there.* Personal decision on my part.

Debra's
BRACHA.org.il

I proceeded to have a prophylactic bilateral mastectomy with a DIEP reconstruction. This was a microsurgery that took a flap of fat from my stomach and placed it into breast mounds created by a skin-sparing mastectomy. I have no regrets whatsoever and am very pleased with the physical outcome.

About six months after, I had a prophylactic hysterectomy and the recovery was easy, because I had it done laparoscopically. Again, I had no regrets.

I now feel completely at ease and well to go on and lead my life. I realize that even in the passing/death of my father, he gave me the blessing, the blessing of life. (Bracha is the Hebrew word for blessing.)

Amy S.
Sister Was Diagnosed in Her Thirties

I look at my sister, who was in her early thirties when she was diagnosed with breast cancer and is now dying of both breast and ovarian cancer, in her late thirties.

My sister tells me all the time that if she had known we had this genetic flaw, she'd have done everything in her power to avoid cancer. She is my strongest backer of my upcoming surgeries. I am having a hysterectomy and bilateral mastectomy in January.

I feel guilty I have this choice at my sister's misfortune. She has told me that at least something positive is coming out of her cancer. I have my sister to thank for bearing this burden of cancer to save my life.

Jackie M.
Get it Together!

The biggest problem I've had is coordination of care. If we want to get certain procedures and tests done, we don't necessarily know where to go. Help us figure it out. It's really helpful to have someone who is part of the system help us wade through the logistical stuff.

Also, don't try to downplay the risks. My GP told me, "Remember, that's an eighty-seven-percent chance over your whole life." Actually, only until age seventy, and I plan to live past seventy, but never mind that. Uh, that's still pretty bad. While that means my doctor will probably never see me get breast cancer, I will probably see me get breast cancer if I don't get a mastectomy.

Lisa Grocott
Bad Experiences

My most negative experience was getting a mammo before my surgery. One of the technicians made a big fuss about the fact I was having a prophylactic mastectomy. She clearly was uninformed, but the best part was that my doctor immediately said she wouldn't use that place any more and rescheduled my other imaging to another facility.

Teri

Lisa, you reminded me of when I went in for my one and only breast MRI, before my PBM. The initial technician, when taking my vital signs, asked me why I was having an MRI. She knew nothing about BRCA mutations. When I told her I was about to have a PBM, her jaw dropped and she said, "But you're so young! Are you sure you want to do that?"

Oh, and for my hyst/ooph, the morning of my surgery, as I was in my hospital gown getting prepped, one of the nurses said to me: "You know after this surgery you won't be able to have any more children, right?" And then she also made reference to my young age. Um, hi there! Do I have a stupid sign on my head?

First of all, I'm not as young as I look! So thank you. Secondly, yes, I know what I'm doing, I've thought about it, in fact, have thought of little else the past year! So frustrating.

Oophorectomy/Hysterectomy

Teri's Blog
FU to BRCA1 (2009)

So October will come, and I'll have the surgery. Yes, I'll go through instant menopause, which I'm sure will be awful, but it beats getting ovarian cancer, going through chemotherapy, and having death hang over my head like an ill-tempered storm cloud. It means that I win. It means that I took this genetic test, found this scientific crystal ball, and I get to change the course of my life for the better.

I don't have to be like my mother who is now battling ovarian cancer. I don't have to be like one of her sisters, who lost her battle to ovarian cancer, or like my grandmother, who during her autopsy was found with ovarian cancer, or like any of those others who battled this disease. That won't be me, because I have the ability to circumvent all of that. I win!

So FU to you, BRCA1 predisposition to hereditary cancers! In your face.

Jenny D.
What My Oncologist Says

My oncologist says that, to this day, he will sleep better once I have my oophorectomy done.

Dr. Herman

Teri was spot on when she blogged about her BSO. Additional portions of those blog posts are included in this book. Also, take specific notice of Dr. Sheila K.'s personal story of how she was saved via BRCA testing.

On Removal of Ovaries and Fallopian Tubes

It is important to always remember that whenever you discuss removal of the ovaries, you must be sure to point out to your patients that it's both the ovaries and fallopian tubes (BSO or bilateral salpingo-oopherectomy). Twenty to thirty percent of what we originally thought were ovarian cancers, we have learned actually originated in the fallopian tubes.

Dr. Sheila K.
BRCA Testing Saved My Life

My father's first cousins, when they found out they were BRCA positive, made it their mission to tell the entire family about having the BRAC1 gene. Because of them, I went and got tested. I believe that BRCA testing saved my life. I tested positive, too, and decided to undergo prophylactic surgery to remove my ovaries. They actually found I had ovarian cancer before I became symptomatic.

My surgery was a complete success, and I have completed six cycles of chemotherapy. I was maintained on Avastin[27] every three weeks and today, eighteen months after receiving the diagnosis, my scans are good, my markers remain normal, and I am feeling great!

Many ovarian cancers are found after months of symptoms when it has already spread past the pelvis (mine was found before it spread). I consider myself lucky and am very grateful to my cousins!

Thanks for doing what needed to be done.

Dr. Herman
On Never Finding Early Ovarian Cancer

Dear Dr. K., Many OB/GYNs in their entire career never find early invasive ovarian cancer. Your BRCA story and your cousins' action should inspire the rest of us. We all need to be more proactive and get the appropriate people tested. More people need to hear your story.

Teri
On Getting Rid Of the Dark Cloud

After going to a Facing our Risk of Cancer Empowered (FORCE) meeting, and seeing and meeting the women who had gone through with it, who had their oophorectomy and PBM and reconstruction, I couldn't help but notice their sense of happiness. They don't have to live with a dark cloud over their heads every day.

Teri's Blog
Patients and Staff Don't Know Medical Terminology

There is a lot of terminology involved once you start breaking it down. It seems like not even a lot of medical professionals know the exact wording. The last time I gave my medical history to the nurse at my OB/GYN's office, she said, "You had a hysterectomy, right?"

I said, "Yes, and an oophorectomy."

She responded, "Oh, okay, so you had a total hysterectomy." I didn't bother to correct her, but in hindsight, maybe I should have.

As a medical practitioner, you should make sure your patients understand what you are talking about but also that your staff is educated as well.

Copy, print and hand this out to your staff for memorization:

Hysterectomy: *the removal of the uterus*

Subtotal or partial hysterectomy: *removal of the fundus or top portion of the uterus*

Complete hysterectomy: *both the uterus and the cervix are removed*

Radical hysterectomy: *the removal of the uterus, cervix, ovaries, tubes, lymph nodes, and surrounding tissues to the sidewalls*

Salpingo-oophorectomy: *removal of an ovary and fallopian tube*

Bilateral salpingo-oophorectomy (BSO): *removal of both ovaries and both fallopian tubes.*

Total Abdominal Hysterectomy and Bilateral Salpingo-Oophorectomy (TAH-BSO): *a total abdominal hysterectomy and bilateral salpingo-oophorectomy performed as one procedure*

Prophylactic: *When used before oophorectomy or mastectomy it relates to the preventative aspect. It means the removal of healthy organs and tissue. If surgery removes cancer-ridden ovaries, tubes and/or breasts, it wouldn't be prophylactic.*

Maria
Should I Have a Hysterectomy, Too?

Dear Teri and Dr. Herman: My question is, *What advice can you give me on keeping the uterus or not?* It has been recommended to me that I remove my ovaries and tubes but there is no need to take the uterus.

Now, I'm interested in hearing your opinions about that. I feel like it should ultimately be my decision and not my gynecologist's, but it is not easy to find information that is very helpful. So now I turn to you. Give me some advice, please!

Teri's Blog
Hysterectomy and Oophorectomy

Maria, when I first learned I'd need to have my ovaries taken out to avoid my high risk of ovarian cancer, I was told that I needed to decide if I wanted to have a hysterectomy, too. What were they talking about? Should I have a hysterectomy too or just the oophorectomy? It can all be very confusing!

Before my surgery I asked my GYN/ONC for her opinion. She's a genetics expert and knows everything there is to know about BRCA-related cancers. She advised me to have all of it removed. "Why?" I asked. "As a BRCA1 positive woman, am I more prone to uterine and cervical cancer, too?"

The answer was no, but she still told me to have my uterus taken out. I left my appointment more confused than ever. I came home and saw my local OB/GYN, who gave me the same answers. He thought I should have it all removed, even though I wasn't more prone to uterine and cervical cancer. This didn't make a lot of sense to me, but these people were in the know. I trusted their judgment. Even so, I started digging deeper before I made my decision.

"Just because" wasn't a compelling reason for me. I remember feeling overwhelmed and confused by this in the beginning. I didn't understand the point of having a hysterectomy when my risk of uterine cancer and cervical cancer was no more than anyone else's. After more searching, I learned that there are good reasons to consider it.

Dr. Herman
On Deciding on a Hysterectomy & Oophorectomy

Agreed. Most studies indicate there is no increased risk of uterine or cervical cancer for the BRCA positive woman in comparison to everyone else. This is why, as of today, a hysterectomy is not part of the recommendations. So why do some women have it done?

There are two main medical reasons. Removing ovaries and tubes for a young woman results in premature menopause. Hot flashes, night sweats, vaginal dryness, loss of libido are just a few of the exciting menopausal symptoms. Many women request relief of the symptoms with hormone replacement. Well, that may be a problem as the WHI study reports[28] that taking estrogen and progesterone hormone replacement for significant periods increases the risk of breast cancer. On the bright side, they also report taking estrogen alone, without added progesterone, showed no increase in breast cancer risk.

Why is progesterone added to the estrogen? Because of the effect of estrogen on the uterus. Estrogen causes the uterine lining to grow. Hyperplasia and/or cancer may result if nothing is done to stop the unopposed growth. Progesterone is that opposition. So, progesterone stops uterine cancer but may help cause some additional breast cancers.

All these years, we've thought estrogen caused the breast cancer when it really was the progesterone. *The butler did it! The butler did it!* But really it was the maid. If one is considering hormone replacement, take out the uterus at the time of BSO so estrogen alone can be given for menopausal relief.

The second reason to take out the uterus is if a patient plans on the use of chemo-preventive medication to reduce the risk of breast cancer. One of Tamoxifen's side effects is endometrial (uterine) cancer. If your patient doesn't have a uterus, then she cannot get uterine cancer. So the second good reason to have the uterus removed at the time of BSO.

I have heard from a number of patients that they had their uterus removed because their doctor told them to do it as long as they were there anyway. Not such a good reason. Our patients deserve real answers to this question.

I have also heard of patients requesting the uterus and cervix be removed because they fear they will get cancer if it is left behind. Also, not the best reason but I can understand the request. With correct information, women will be able make educated choices.

Tips for Performing a BRCA BSO

From One Doctor to Another

- *Consent patient for possible laparotomy and full-staging procedure. There's a small but real chance cancer will be found.*
- *Let the GYN/ONC know you are doing the case in the event that you find cancer and need their help. A little heads up type of thing.*
- *Take peritoneal washings.*
- *Look at the omentem, liver, and diaphragm.*
- *Take the entire tube and ovary on each side.*
- *Burn the cornua to destroy any remaining tube remnant.*
- *Write BRCA in big letters on the pathology request form.*
- *Call pathologist and remind them to cut the pathology specimen properly; i.e., a detailed evaluation of the entire specimen, 2-3mm slices.*

Teri's Blog
On Tamoxifen and Side Effects

I researched the side effects of Tamoxifen. In my mind, there are a number of reasons why I personally wouldn't want to be on it. To name a few: Tamoxifen increases risk of osteoporosis. Guess what? So does an oophorectomy. So it'd be a double whammy risk of osteoporosis.

Tamoxifen increases the risk of blood clots (pulmonary embolism, deep vein thrombosis, strokes). Yep, yep, and for people like me, who've already had a blood clot and pulmonary embolism, I personally know that is a very frightening side effect and one that could lead to death if not diagnosed and treated quickly. I'd rather avoid adding another risk factor into my life.

Some less serious side effects are: Some people call it Tamoxifen brain (it's much like chemo brain). It can negatively affect the memory. Oophorectomy can do the same.

Libido: many breast cancer patients who are on Tamoxifen report a decrease in their libido. Also a very likely side effect of the oophorectomy. Tamoxifen is sometimes used on sex offenders, as a form of chemical castration. Scary!

Lest I sound like I'm all anti-Tamoxifen, I'd like to point out there are some good side effects, too. It can prevent breast cancer in some patients, including those of us who are at high risk of getting breast cancer. As you are aware, it's used to treat active cases of breast cancer, in both women and men.

Would I want to trade my risk of breast cancer just to get a risk of something else that may be just as bad? Obviously, for me, the answer was no. For some people though, the answer is yes. That doesn't mean they are wrong, and I am right. Just different perspectives.

We all deserve the right to make our own choices. We can make better choices if we have all of the correct information.

Jenny D.
BSO Is for Me, Despite the Risks

I know the right choice for me is a prophylactic oophorectomy. I know my risks. It's weird to say that. I know my risk increases for cardiovascular disease, decreased libido, etc. but I want to live to experience or to not experience and to just live to see another day to make all different kinds of choices. Most importantly, to watch my children do the same. I have to. I lost my mom. I don't want my kids to have that feeling of being cheated. I have to be here, so the parts have to leave.

Teri's Blog
I Scheduled My BSO: June 18, 2009

I had officially scheduled my appointment for my hysterectomy and oophorectomy for October 9, 2009. Three days before my thirty-ninth birthday. My pre-operative appointment was September 29. When I posted that information on my blog, I received so many comments, emails, and Facebook communication from family and friends that it almost overwhelmed me. I felt so much care, love, and support. The morning I wrote this blog post I started thinking about the upcoming surgery, and I felt positively giddy about it. Maybe it was writing and getting all of my feelings out there. Maybe it was the outpouring of positive energy flowing my way.

Maybe it's my sweet, loving family, always standing by me. More likely it's a combination of all of those things. I felt so strong all of a sudden. I felt like standing up on the table, sticking out my tongue, and shouting, "Take that, BRCA1!"

I felt like I was taking my power back again. I was regaining power over my own destiny, my life.

Teri's Blog
Burning Tampons

Leading up to the surgery, I went out with some close friends with the intention of having a Tampon Burning Party. A friend of mine, Bryn, had originally suggested it, earlier on. At the time, I was actually silently mortified at the idea, and even hurt my feelings that a good friend of mine would joke about something so serious. But after a few months, the idea grew on me. The more I thought about it, the more I knew I had to have a party like that.

A red velvet cake made to look just like a tampon box was made in my honor. We had a good time, drinking and laughing. We shared stories of how cancer had touched our lives. I felt comforted by the support. I am not sure if they even know how much it meant to me that they took a few hours out of their busy lives to be there with me, helping me to blow off some steam and interject a little humor into a very serious subject that had consumed my thoughts since I learned of my BRCA1 mutation. It meant the world to me to have them there.

The entire time, I never knew for sure if I would actually burn any tampons. I brought a box with me just in case. When the night was coming to a close I decided to just do it. I like the symbolism behind it. We gathered our purses and stepped outside. I handed each friend a tampon.

We stood in a circle. I lit the first one and then one by one the rest of the tampons were added to the bonfire. We laughed. We joked. Some of my friends wished it were their tampons that we were burning. Being rid of the dreaded monthly cycle didn't sound so bad to them. I laughed along with them. The reasons for my surgery were very clear in my mind. I was doing it to save my life.

The night ended with a tampon bonfire. Yes, we really did light tampons on fire and watched them burn.

So the next day, the morning after, I felt hung over for sure but I also felt good. I'm glad I had the party and said my farewells to the parts of me that brought me two wonderful sons. I was grateful for the support of my loving husband, who waited half-asleep on the couch for me to get home that night. I am happy and thankful to have such caring friends. I'm glad for the silver lining.

I'm on the Way: October 7, 2009

I wrote this the evening before leaving home for my (BSO/hyst) surgery. We live so far from Cedars Sinai that we have had to stay in a hotel the night before. I had to be in the hospital at 5:15a.m. on Friday morning for surgery at 7:15a.m.

Surgery. My surgery--a hysterectomy and oophorectomy.

I had been thinking about it for so long by then. Okay, to say *thinking* is to put it mildly. I had been dwelling on it for so long, it was weird for it to be looming so close.

I Skyped with my BRCA1-positive friend, Karen Malkin-Lazarovitz, or Karen from Canada, as I fondly call her, earlier that morning. She had already gone through it. She assured me, as many others who have gone before me do, that when I woke up from surgery it will be with a huge sense of relief. As

I bid farewell to my ovaries, fallopian tubes, uterus, and cervix, I also got to say goodbye to my forty four percent chance of ovarian cancer. Forty-four percent. Forty. Four. Percent.

That's good news, super good news. So I'm not really sure why I felt like I wanted to puke that night. Sorry for my lack of eloquence.

The Day of Surgery: October 9, 2009

When I arrived at Cedars Sinai at 5:15a.m., I almost immediately felt frustrated. The girl who checked me in was about as rude and unfeeling as a person could be. My annoyance grew while I thought about it. People go into surgery nervous as it is. My opinion is that the first point of contact at the hospital should think about that and try to at least be nice to incoming patients. It was just as if the human factor were forgotten. She was all business, just trying to get through the waiting room full of people, no smiles, no well wishes, just *wham* *bam*, thank you, ma'am, and next.

The orderly who came to collect me was almost as bad. I felt my heart rate quicken and my anger rise. I felt much like cattle being herded or a convict in prison. I couldn't believe it.

Once I got behind the double doors, some of the people I came in contact with seemed to get nicer at least. The anesthesiologist was very friendly and did his best to explain to me what was going on and what to expect.

After I asked the nurse about five times, they finally brought Travis back to me. I needed his calming influence so much! I was scared and nervous and as he walked up to me tears openly poured out of my eyes, down my face. He stood there caressing my leg as a group of doctors and surgical nurses came over to introduce themselves.

Dr. Karlan walked up too, beaming a big, reassuring smile at me. The anesthesia must have then taken effect because the next thing I remembered was waking up in the recovery room.

As of Friday, October 9, at approximately 10:30ish, my risk of ovarian cancer was downgraded to less than two percent.

Voices from the Crowd

Pat Martin
What If?

I knew from the start I would get the surgeries. I am scheduled for my BSO next week and the breasts will follow soon. I have had my moments of being so thankful to have the news to crying like a baby. I can't help at times to ask myself, "What if I had been diagnosed with cancer before now?"

Lulu Luke
Family Tree

Since finding out I have the mutation I have traced the family tree on my dad's side and, although there are no other breast cancers, there is a second cousin related to me through unaffected males who died from ovarian cancer at forty-five. That made me decide to have my ovaries taken out. So I had a TAH/BSO.

Pam W.
Hot Flashes

The first couple months the hot flashes were happening all the time (plus it was summertime so that didn't help matters much). But six months later, in the dead of winter, I rarely have any hot flashes! It's freezing here! Where are the hot flashes when you need them! *Ha!*

Karen Malkin-Lazarovitz
Take it All

I'm on .05 of Climara[29] and have been since my hysterectomy in February 2009. I had everything removed: ovaries, fallopian tubes, uterus, and cervix. I am one-hundred percent confident with my decision and feel great.

I chose to have my uterus removed for three reasons:

1. *I don't need it anymore.*
2. *I don't want to take progesterone.*
3. *One less type of cancer to worry about.*

Helen Smith
Glad I Did It

I had my surgery done laparoscopically. I had all my parts removed, as I didn't need them and didn't want to risk cervical cancer, either. I had a dysplasia on my cervix when I was eighteen. I am on .075 Vivelle dot for my HRT. I am glad that I had it done. I was back to work in six days.

Lisa Edwards

I figure, if you aren't going to use it, get rid of it.

Menopause and More
On Hormone Replacement Therapy

Teri's Blog
Plunging into Menopause

When a woman has her ovaries removed, it plunges her into instant surgical menopause. As a woman, I've always dreaded knowing menopause would eventually be something I'd go through, just like every other woman. This is such a common fear among females! We've all seen the crazed menopausal woman depicted in film or TV and none of us want to be like that. The idea of being out of control of our emotions is frightening!

Hearing we might lose our sexual urges is also a big concern. Studies show that often the symptoms of surgical menopause are much more severe than for those who arrive at menopause naturally.[30] In addition to that, the younger a woman is when having this surgery, typically the worse her symptoms are.

Possible Symptoms of Menopause

- *Hot flashes*
- *Irritability and mood swings*
- *Night sweats*
- *Hair loss*
- *Insomnia*
- *Vaginal dryness*
- *Weight gain*

- *Decrease in sexual desire*
- *Loss of cognitive (typically memory) abilities*

As if the above weren't enough already, I read that it probably increases the likelihood of developing heart disease and osteoporosis. Studies also show that surgical menopause may also heighten the risk of lung cancer, especially for those who don't take estrogen therapy.[31]

Some doctors tell their patients who are having a hysterectomy that it will cause bladder prolapse while some say that it's simply a myth and just not true. The simple solution to avoid dealing with symptoms associated with menopause is to go on hormone replacement therapy (HRT) or estrogen replacement therapy (ERT), if this is an option (individual cases will vary).

Some doctors refuse the use of HRT of any kind for BRCA-positive women. In my mind, this is a shortsighted view. Quality of life issues are important and must be considered on a case-by-case basis.

Teri's Blog
On Hot Flashes

My ovaries are out. Rough night sleeping last night as I tossed and turned with night sweats. I woke up this morning to the never-ending hot flash. It was about four hours long. If you've never had a hot flash, the best way for me to describe it is as if someone has taken one of those high voltage portable heaters and put it on the inside of your body. I was so desperate for some relief, I stripped my clothes off and blasted the cooler. So the outside of my body became cold, goosebumps and everything, but the inside of my body continued to feel like it was on fire.

Honestly, as if periods weren't bad enough? We finally get rid of those, and have to go through menopause? WTF, Mother Nature? What did we ever do to you?

Instant surgical menopause is even worse because we don't get to ease into it. I've been a basket case. For a few days, I thought things were settling down, but no, I was wrong. My friend, Rian from the UK, swears by sticking magnets in her knickers, and I'm desperate enough I'm going to give it a try.

Magnets. In my underwear. Who would have thought?

WHI Findings

While I was at my post-op follow-up appointment for my TAH/BSO, I used some of my time to question my GYN/ONC, Dr. Beth Karlan, and her nurse, Paula Anastasia, up one end and down the other about estrogen therapy. According to the Women's Health Initiative (WIH) study, the amount of estrogen a woman receives through an estrogen patch is so small (between .05 to .1 ml) that it does not increase the risk of breast cancer.

I asked Dr. Karlan how much estrogen our body produces naturally, and she told me that it makes about ten times the amount received by the estrogen patch, about one milligram. This is also when I learned it's not just our ovaries that create estrogen, though those are the main estrogen producers.

According to Dr. Karlan and other well-respected doctors, such as Dr. Steven Narod of Canada (he started the longest running BRCA study around), there are very few reasons for a woman to suffer the effects of menopause. The amount of estrogen released into our bodies from the patch after the oophorectomy and hysterectomy is enough to help us avoid menopausal symptoms but not so much that it will do anything to increase our risk of breast cancer.

Discussing Hormone Therapy before BSO

Some things we just don't know until after we have our surgery, such as how badly this surgically-induced, instant menopause will affect us individually. It's all fine and dandy to decide we don't care about hormone replacement therapy (HRT) or estrogen replacement therapy (ERT) before we are in the midst of dealing with full-blown effects of menopause. It's hard to make a decision based on facts we won't have until after our surgery. So please don't forget to talk to your patients about it.

Yes, menopause sounds awful, and I can't say I look forward to dealing with any of it at the age of thirty-nine. Ovarian cancer has been the killer in my family. My mother is battling it now.

Anyway, with the high risk in my family, and the hormone issue, for me, it was the right choice to have both the hysterectomy and the oophorectomy.

Some Doctors Always Say No

Allowing a woman who is at a high risk of breast cancer to use estrogen therapy is a hot topic. Some doctors won't allow it and some will. Some women are afraid of it and refuse to use it, whether it is doctor approved or not.

I posted a simple question on my Facebook page one day. My query was: "Estrogen therapy: yea or nay?" It got many responses in record time.

Voices from the Crowd

Rachel H.
Such a Hard One

Right now, I'm three weeks out of surgery and even with my patch I'm dealing with lots of symptoms. Our mutation is such a scary thing. We do so much to prevent getting cancer and yet the thing we use to help us get through the day after our surgery could put us dealing with the same thing we went through all those surgeries to avoid.

Bonnie Golden

Estrogen? Nay. Phytoestrogens? Nay. Bring on the night sweats, hot flashes, etc., etc., and memory loss as well!

Elisa

So far I feel pretty fine most of the time. I take supplements, DIM supplements. Also half a dose of Estrotone (which has black cohosh). For joint pain, I take tart cherry. So far all of these things work for me. Also exercise and a good diet helps, too. I know supplements aren't one-hundred-percent safe, but my personal opinion is they are safer than synthetic hormones. Just my opinion, not medical fact.

Tara Beirens

I haven't had surgery yet but will in a couple of months and I am totally yay for estrogen. I do not want to be a crazy person. From what I understand, it doesn't raise my risk all that much.

Elaine W.
Yay for Me

I am four weeks post-op and my OB/GYN put me on Premarin[32] (with permission from my oncologist), after I visited her office for my first post-op hot flash and crying like a child. I've been through chemo and the way I felt that day made me want to die, just like chemo did (of course chemo was way worse). I figure, since I have no real breasts anymore, it's worth any risk. Before the HRT, I felt like I had jumped off a cliff. Kudos to you, ladies who go it alone. Seriously, my hat off to you.

Teri's Blog
The Last Word on My TAH/BSO

I wrote that five months after surgery. All the stuff I worried about, it's over: the surgery, the recovery, the forty-four-percent risk of ovarian cancer... done.

I dreaded instant menopause, but it wasn't initially a problem. Yes, I had a few hot flashes, but only at night. Honestly, they hadn't been that big of a deal, except for the initial recovery time.

Do I regret having the surgery? Of course not! Not for a minute! The pain from surgery and recovery is temporary; BRCA-type cancer is not. In fact, with its high reoccurrence rate, it's anything but temporary and is not something I want to mess around with, obviously!

Sex and Sexuality after BSO

Teri's Blog: November 7, 2009

This section contains talk of a sexual nature. If you are easily offended, you might want to pass on reading this. If you are my son, brother, relative, or my dad, I'm serious; don't read this!

I wrote this when I was one month post-op from my TAH/BSO. The fatigue and soreness in my stomach are gone. I think I'd be safe saying I feel recovered from surgery.

A question that has been asked on Facebook and my blog several times now is about libido after BSO. I've also seen this question posted on message boards time and time again. A lot of women fear that when their ovaries are gone, they will turn into dried up, non-sexually minded, ugly, old hags. Not my words, I've actually heard and read people say this. Many fear their urge for sex will be gone, as will their body's ability to create natural lubrication. Some women are worried their orgasms will change. They fear sex will be "less" than it was before. They worry that the spark inside them will be gone.

As of four weeks ago, I have no ovaries, fallopian tubes, uterus, or cervix. I am using an estrogen patch that gives me a teeny amount of estrogen to help avoid the menopause symptoms.

I don't feel like less of a woman. I don't feel dried up, ugly, or haggish. As a matter of fact, my husband thinks I'm damned sexy, and there are times I even agree with him.

After surgery like this, it is advised to refrain from sexual intercourse for four to six weeks. There are internal stitches and a lot of healing that needs to go on before having sex. Travis and I have had the hardest (no pun intended) time waiting. I'm here to clear the air and dismiss your patient's worries: My libido did not disappear with my reproductive organs. I'm still as hot for Travis as I've always been, and he is for me. We spent the past four weeks making out like teenagers with no below the belt action (for me, anyway).

Yesterday being the four-week mark, we decided to go for it. I wanted to take it slow, fearing it might hurt. Have you ever made love slowly? It was intense. It didn't hurt. Natural lubrication was not a problem for me. Things got more and more heated. We were in our own little world and we climaxed together. My orgasm was just as strong as it ever was. When we were done, I had a racing heart and had to catch my breath. It was wonderful.

Losing my reproductive organs did not change who I am as a person. It didn't make me less sexy or less sexual. For women, sexual excitement doesn't always begin in the private parts or reproductive organs anyway. It begins in the mind. For me, it starts when I glance up and notice Travis looking at me with that certain gleam in his eye. I know what he's thinking. He's thinking of me... naked. It makes me think of stuff, too. Foreplay gets the juices flowing and by the time he actually penetrates me, I'm already almost over the top. He teases my mind first, then my body.

I think if you have a loving relationship and a good sex life before surgery, you will afterward, too. Breathe easy, sisters, and worry about one less thing.

Teri's Blog: Update January 23, 2010

It's been close to four months now since I had my TAH/BSO.
Everything stated above still holds true. Sex drive is as good as
ever. The first month after surgery I was using an estrogen
patch, Climara .1 ml. Since then, I've been on Climara .05, and
my BSO hasn't affected my sexuality at all.

Voices from the Crowd

Dee
November 8, 2009

Hey Teri, thank you so much for your candor. This is definitely a big issue for me and one of the main reasons I just haven't
been able to sign on for the oophorectomy that all the docs say
I have to get ASAP. Your experience is very reassuring. You're
gorgeous, by the way. Travis is one lucky guy!

Teri to Dee
November 8, 2009

You aren't the only one, Dee. I've met so many women who
are terrified of losing their sexuality along with their ovaries. It
was hard for me to hit the "publish" button on this one. I have
no anonymity at all, but I truly wanted to alleviate the con-

cerns that so many women have. I honestly think that if you are a sexual creature before menopause, then you will be one afterwards, too. And thanks for the compliment. That's so sweet.

Lita Poehlman (Teri's Maternal Aunt)
November 7, 2009

Dear Teri, I told you so! Yes, sisters, at sixty-eight with a complete hysterectomy, I still feel the same on the inside. Love you so much.

Kathi
November 7, 2009

The thing is, though, I think some of us are just extra libidinous. Which is just plain luck, I think. I know lots of women who do have trouble with their mojo and their juices for all kinds of reasons. But I'm one of those women also whose libido never seems to be affected by anything that is supposed to dry it and me right up. Peri-menopause? Nah. Post-menopause? Nah. Antidepressants? Nah. Having half my boob cut off? Nah. What can I say?

I'm not sure we're the norm, though, but perhaps we can at least represent a bit of reassurance to those who have been told that it's a foregone conclusion that you need a big pile of estrogen to be libidinous. Actually, for women, it's our little pile of testosterone (yes, we do have some of that, too) that probably makes more of a difference.

Barbara
April 11, 2010

I am here to say I am a Previvor! I had my hysterectomy four years ago, and I agree, sexuality is a state of mind. With the right foreplay, it's on.

The body is a wonderful thing. I experienced full menopause instantly after surgery and opted not to use estrogen patches, although the flashes were a bit of a hurdle. The intensity of the change was not gradual, but once it's over, it's over.

The message to other women: Put your fears aside! Part of the pro-active stance you took in having preventative surgeries applies to everything else. It's about doing all you can: oils, lotions, and a creative mind will still do the job! Eat right, exercise helps a lot, and keep a smile on because the best is yet to cum! (Sorry for the indiscretion.) Stay strong. Stay positive and surrounded by those you love that support you!

Elaine
October 29, 2010

Well, Teri, my girlie-parts' days are numbered now. December 6th is the date the time bombs will depart from this body. My wonderful boyfriend will be here to bid them *adieu*.

I've always been a sexual being, and I was foolish to think that getting my ovaries removed would affect what was in my mind. These are things I knew all along, but sometimes you listen to horror stories some women tell. I think these stories come from women who probably didn't have a strong libido to begin with and perhaps trying to please their husbands after the surgery was more of a chore or a nightmare for them. I'm definitely not worried about it any more and look forward to this being the last thing I'll have to do for the BRCA1 mutation.

Cathy
June 15, 2010

Dear Teri, thank you for sharing your story. You made me feel better just reading it. Since having my laparoscopically assisted vaginal hysterectomy (LAVH), I somehow felt less of a woman. Can't explain it. I started losing interest in all things important, my horse riding, for one thing, constantly thinking my insides would fall out or something. Anyway, your story has made me feel one-hundred percent better!

Teri
November 8, 2009

It was a little scary to share that entry, but I honestly wanted to show that menopause (surgical or otherwise) isn't (doesn't have to be) the end of (sex) life.

2013

Well, here I am, a few years later, and I hate to say it, but I have to say it. While I was able to use the estrogen patch, my sex life was great. I was forced to ditch it after I developed a DVT and PEs as a result of traveling on an airplane after one of my reconstruction surgeries.

Since being off the patch, things are more difficult in that department. My libido has taken a definite nosedive. I've been actively trying to help it along though. All hope is not lost. Once I do let myself get in the mood, then it can still be good! Though, in all honesty, it takes more work now than it used to.

Pre-prophylactic Bilateral Mastectomy & Reconstruction

Teri's Blog
I Decided on a Mastectomy: One

Initially, I had mostly made up my mind that I'd have my fallopian tubes and ovaries removed, but never my breasts. After talking with people who actually know what's up, I changed my mind. I think for me, removing my ovaries and removing my breasts, while scary as all hell, was a less-scary alternative than having the big eighty-seven-percent risk looming over my head. After all, I am not my insides; I am not my breasts; I am me.

I'd rather be minus a few parts than battle cancer, especially this type of aggressive take-no-prisoners type of cancer or to constantly worry and wonder my whole life when I'm going to get it, not if! It will come back, if I've already battled and beaten it.

Teri's Blog
I Decided on a Mastectomy: Two

After I learned I was a BRCA1 mutation carrier it didn't take much research for me to find out that the best course of action to avoid cancer was to have a prophylactic bilateral mastectomy (PBM) and prophylactic bilateral salpingo-oopherectomy.

In the early days, before learning all that I know now, I was terrified. I'd always loved the shape and size of my breasts. Even though they are on the smaller side, I still think they are quite pretty. Perkiness has never been a problem and I'd never, ever considered implants. Those were just not my style. Thinking that I had to make a choice of waiting around for cancer to strike versus sacrificing my breasts had me in a world of turmoil in those early days.

I kept imagining myself in my bathroom, standing in front of the mirror, naked after taking a shower. In this twisted daydream, I'd stare into my reflection and see my chest area devoid of breasts and covered with scars from end to end, mutilated. A lump would form in my throat, and I'd do my best to shake the picture from my mind. No matter how hard I'd try, over and over it would pop back in. I would cry at the drop of a hat and beat myself up for being so vain; after all, at least I had a chance to avoid this horrible, aggressive type cancer that follows BRCA mutations. Having my breasts sliced off is surely better than dying.

I started to educate myself more. I then learned that these days a mastectomy is usually followed by reconstruction. I had thought at first that the only reconstruction options were implants. I didn't much care for this idea. As I'd mentioned, I was pretty happy with my breasts as they were and never imagined myself as an implant type of girl.

More weeks passed, and I did even more research on breast reconstruction. I found an option that sounded right up my alley.

It's called a DIEP flap and it stands for deep inferior epigastric perforator. It takes tummy fat (and no, you don't have to have a ton of extra fat to do it, just enough) and the new breasts are recreated from that. It gives you a very natural look. The breasts lose and gain weight as you do, and I get a tummy tuck along with it. I'm not a big girl, but have always had this little pooch of fat that I've never been able to do anything about. It was there even when I was a waifish ninety-nine pounds. I decided I was going with the DIEP.

There are many different types of flap tissue breast reconstruction options, such as:[33]

DIEP: Deep Inferior Epigastric Perforator

In a nutshell, the DIEP uses the body's own tummy fat and skin to rebuild, or reconstruct the breasts. No muscle is cut, but it is microsurgery, as blood vessels have to be reattached. On the plus side, a tummy tuck is included as part of the procedure.

TRAM: Transverse Rectus Abdominis Muscle

Very similar to the DIEP, but the stomach muscles are cut quite badly and the recovery time is a lot longer and harder than DIEP.

S-GAP: Superior Gluteal Artery Perforator

Fat and skin is taken from the upper buttock and used to reconstruct the breasts. No muscles are cut with this tissue procedure either, and it, like the DIEP, is considered to be microsurgery.

I-GAP: Inferior Gluteal Artery Perforator

This procedure is the same as above, but it uses fat and skin from the lower buttock instead of the upper.

SIEA: Superficial Inferior Epigastric Artery Flap

This flap procedure is almost the same as DIEP, except the blood vessels are taken from just under the surface of the lower abdomen.

TUG: Inner Thigh Flap

This procedure is usually used by very thin or athletic women, or women who may have had previous abdominoplasty. This procedure is becoming more common in the United States.

Question from the BRCA Sisterhood Group on Facebook:

What is the process of finding the best breast surgeon and plastic surgeon?

Teri
I Made a List

When I decided on surgery, I started by coming up with a list of doctors who can do the mastectomy/reconstruction. I'd had to check out several before taking action. I was being so cautious about my decision-making, which is not my normal mode of operation. But it is my life I'm talking about here, and my body parts, and I didn't want to just pick the first doctor I saw or heard about.

Angela S.
Be Informed

A lot of doctors don't know what information is right, up to date, etc., and as patients, we trust their decisions. It's hard when we are trying to look for answers and stuff.

When I first called a surgeon to see if I could schedule a consultation for a prophylactic bilateral mastectomy, due to a BRCA mutation, nobody at that doctor's office knew what I was talking about. I decided I probably should not go to that particular doctor. It's sad that even doctors don't know what's up and the information you read on the internet isn't always reliable, either. It's frustrating!

Teri
Experience and Rapport

I wanted to go to someone who has done hundreds of these surgeries. I wanted to have a good rapport with him/her. I didn't want to stress out over things that could go wrong during all of this. I think maybe it's okay I screeched to a halt in the process like I did, to give myself time to absorb it all, to learn, to talk to others, to think about it, to write about it, to be making this decision. I know, while the idea of chopping off my healthy breasts was terrifying, it was my best option at this time.

Dr. Herman
Learning Who's Who

As a gynecologist, I made it my business to meet all the breast surgeons and plastic surgeons in my area. I learned about their particular interests and specialties. I didn't understand then that there were so many different kinds of reconstruction options and different surgeons had affinities for certain types. Now, I know. I put together a list with phone numbers and addresses to give to my patients.

I also asked the anesthesiologists and the OR nurses who they would use. No one knows the surgeons better than they do. That worked great. As time went by, I added additional names by speaking with the patients who had reconstruction. I still continue to do so. I find out if the patient is happy with her results, who she used and if she'd use the same surgeon if she had to do it all over again. I try to make sure the type of reconstruction she had is the same one the upcoming patient is considering, or might consider.

Teri's Blog
Losing Sensation

It's truly wonderful what the Center for Restorative Breast Surgery in New Orleans does for women like me.[34] I had my breasts removed and reconstructed and they look very much like the real thing. Honestly, my body will probably end up looking better afterward than it did before. On the downside, I may have lost all feeling in my chest and my stomach may become permanently numb. As positive as I'm trying to keep all of this, I can't fool myself for long by thinking "Yay, tummy tuck and boob job!" It's really not that simple.

My stomach and breast area will lose most, if not all, sensation. I could bump into a wall with my chest and not even realize I did it. I wondered what it will be like when I hug my family or when I'm intimate with my husband.

Update
March 2013

I regained most of my feeling in the areas that were opened up. There are areas of numbness, but it's not something I notice that much.

Dr. Herman

After discussing numbness after reconstruction with Teri, I began asking my patients, and I am happy to report that most of them have had a similar experience as she has. Over time, the numbness has substantially subsided, more than expected.

Angela T.
No Regrets

For your BRCA mutation carriers who are trying to make the tough decision whether to have a prophylactic mastectomy, here is something you might want to consider, but first a little background.

I am a BRCA1 carrier, along with my mother, two sisters, an aunt, and three cousins. Eight of the ten women in my family tested carry the gene. The testing all began because my aunt passed away at thirty-three of breast cancer.

Five and a half years ago (at the age of thirty), I had a mastectomy and months of reconstruction. I have had moments of regret over the years, as I often thought I could have gone with MRIs and mammograms every six months. If something did develop, then they would catch it early. Well, today I am so grateful I made the decision to have the mastectomy! My mother (who is fifty-six years young), was recently diagnosed with triple negative stage I, grade III breast cancer.

As the docs screened her every six months, they caught it early. The problem is, it's a triple negative cancer. My mother has since had a mastectomy and her lymph nodes were clear. She recently started chemo. Why is she doing chemo if her nodes are clear? Because it is triple negative cancer. Because the recurrence rate is twenty to forty percent with no chemo and fifteen to twenty percent with chemo.

Ultimately, the decision is your patients'. I feel so lucky I will not have to worry about getting triple negative breast cancer. And my mom is the most amazing woman I have ever had the pleasure of knowing. Together we are strong and we will beat this thing called cancer.

Dr. Herman

Very good point. From a pathological perspective there has been an increase in triple negative breast cancer with BRCA1 mutations while BRCA2 follows the normal distribution of estrogen positives to triple negatives.

Lisa Marie Guzzardi
I had it Done; My Positive Experience Here

Dear Distinguished Faculty Members, Doctors and Administrators:

It is with profound gratitude and appreciation that I wish to acknowledge my two outstanding surgeons and personalized care during a recent hospitalization at NYU Medical Center.

On the morning of August 10, 2010, I was given a new life, a new beginning with a sense of renewal, hope, and empowerment. I received a priceless gift that was denied to both maternal and paternal grandmothers, aunts and cousins. Each one of these family members suffered from hereditary breast cancer. I refused to become another potential victim of this devastating familial disease.

As a result, I had a risk-reducing bilateral total skin nipple/areola-sparing mastectomy followed by immediate breast reconstruction. Not only does this cutting edge procedure allow many women a dramatic risk reduction, but it also provides us with a huge sense of normalcy and amazing outcomes, without compromising oncological safety. This is also in accordance with the latest research findings that continually demonstrate a broad acceptance and approval within the oncology community. It was the expertise, amazing skill, compassion, and trust with Dr. (redacted) that made this possible for myself. Dr. (redacted) was equally impressive by fully restoring my breasts with such skillful artistry, leaving me with a natural appearance. Together, they have formed a unique and highly skilled partnership. Many women whose lives have been touched by breast cancer, whether they are a Previvor like myself or survivors, have this gentler option. I truly feel as though I have lost nothing, but my risks.

My preoperative, perioperative and postoperative experiences were equally of the highest standards. This journey began in the pre-surgical testing department a week prior to my admission, where all my pre-op concerns were satisfied by the efficiency of a caring nurse practitioner. Upon arrival on 10-East the day of surgery, I was greeted by an RN who completed my pre-op assessment in a soothing professional manner. My attending anesthesiologist explained the protocols of general anesthesia. She made personal allowances for my preferences and wishes. Of course, both attending surgeons provided their ongoing professionalism with the utmost dignified care.

When I entered the operating room, I was warmly welcomed by the entire staff, and I immediately felt safe. During my initial recovery while in the PACU, I found an attentive RN quickly addressing my pain issue, a personal priority need. Later, I was transferred to 12-East for the remainder of my hospitalization. The nursing staff and ancillary staff were all outstanding. I also wish to applaud the integrity of both the surgical oncology and plastics house staff. Their team rounds provided the necessary reassurances and answers I needed regarding my specific care and post-surgical concerns.

From a personal perspective, it is important to recognize the clinical significance of the cancer center. Over the past five years, I was always provided a safe haven for my high-risk surveillance needs, with prevention as the ultimate goal. My previous surgical experiences were focused primarily on early detection, again with the guidance of Dr. Richard Shapiro, a surgical breast oncologist. The comprehensive screenings I received at the diagnostic imaging center through their highly qualified MRI radiology staff were remarkable. The entire fourth floor professional and support staff are recognized as caring individuals. In particular, I am deeply inspired by the unconditional support and outstanding care given by my nurse. She represents the very best of Magnet distinction, an extraordinary example of nursing excellence.

Reflecting upon my long and difficult journey, I am vividly reminded of something I read along the way about NYU Medical Center. *"Excellence is a specialty"* is about delivering the highest quality care at any given moment. To have been a recipient of superior excellence, where I came first, is simply unforgettable and uniquely special!

Dr. Herman to Lisa

Did you actually send this letter to your doctors? Who are your doctors? We all want to know.

Lisa

This is the actual letter I sent to the physicians. My plastic surgeon told me it was one of the nicest letters he had ever received. My surgeons were Dr. Richard Shapiro, breast surgical oncologist and Dr. Nolan Karp of NYU Medical Center.

Teri's Blog
November 10, 2009

My mastectomy was two months and two days away. I still felt mostly calm about it, but once in a while, my heart skipped a beat or two... or twelve. I found myself with my hands on my own breasts a lot. I truly was going to miss them when they were gone. I was not fondling myself, I promise. It's not like that. I just couldn't help but stroke them on occasion, knowing that, very soon, they would be sliced off. *Gulp!* I really shouldn't have put it that way. My heart sped up when I typed the word: *sliced*.

I was going to miss having feeling and sensation on my chest. My breasts have served me well so far. They provided milk, nourishment, and life to my young son for a year. I'm still feeling proud to have met that goal. It may seem like having them cut off is not the best way to show gratitude for all they've done. On the other hand, what better way to show them gratitude than to send them off while they are still somewhat young and lovely? Why take the chance—the up to eighty-seven-percent chance—of letting them be overtaken by cancer? My heart caught in my throat a little bit at that thought. I wondered what it would feel like to hug my family. Man, I was really going to miss my breasts.

Thinking of surgery and recovery was daunting. At that moment, it was more than that that weighed on my mind. It was losing external parts of my body. It was amputation. Yes, they were to be reconstructed, and no one who doesn't see me naked would know the difference. But I'd know the difference. They would have scars. Well, okay, what's one more scar on my body? I have so many anyway. I was rather accident prone in my younger years.

I did my best to keep things on the positive side. I knew a lot of people were reading my blog in those days. They were looking to me for comfort and answers. I've had a lot of comments/messages from people about what a positive attitude I have. But I don't always. I'm human, too. I'm fearful and worried and wish like hell that this wasn't happening to me.

I've repeatedly said the words, "It sucks I have this BRCA1 mutation, but at least I know I have it. It gives me a choice to be proactive." But let's get real here for a minute. Did I really have a choice? What choice was that again? With close to a ninety-percent chance of getting breast cancer, how was having my healthy breasts cut off before cancer strikes really a choice? Deciding between soup or salad, now that's a choice. This? Not so much.

Rissa Watkins
November 10, 2009

Dear Teri, don't worry about needing to be positive for your readers. Mentioning the bad and tearful moments helps people as well. Have I told you yet today how amazing you are? No? Well you are amazing. Even your upset posts have humor and hope. You saved your life by having these surgeries. How many people get to say they are their own hero?

Janine

The nice thing about this surgery is that you will be asleep for the whole thing and when you wake up you will have new stuffing and never see the amputation part. I know some of the numbness will go away after time. I know this woman who showed me her DIEP three months out. She had some feeling and looked fabulous, no nipples and all. I know her scars were not as bad as I thought they would be. And I know she was very happy.

Lita Poehlman
November 12, 2009

Dear Teri, *Hmmm!* Apparently I did harbor some of the feelings you experienced. As I think back before the PBM, I do remember looking at my breasts and touching them more frequently than before making my decision to have the surgery. I was curious about how they would feel. Whether conscious of it or not, we as women, do have a special affinity for our breasts, both for their sexual role in our lives and their nurturing role. Of all our body parts, they do define our sexuality probably the most, but not who we are in heart and spirit.

My doc told me mine would be numb for about a year, so that sounded encouraging, as it indicates some feeling will return over time. This is good news for you young ones! Even if the feeling doesn't come back completely, there are so many other parts of our bodies that are highly sensual, and I'm sure that women can all use their imaginations and creativity so that their lives won't be changed in ways as drastic as you may be thinking pre-surgery!

I keep thinking how very lucky and truly blessed we all are to have the choices we have.

Susan G.

As my surgery approached, my courage grew. My mantra became "I'm going to get the cancer before the cancer gets me." I prepared for surgery according to my doctors' instructions. When I was wheeled into the operating room, I reminded myself that the doctors were not trying to kill me; they were trying to make me well. And I was trying to make me well by saving my life.

Teri Asks

Dr. Herman, do you have any advice you give to women before their mastectomy?

Dr. Herman

I like to tell my patients, get out of the house. Go out to dinner.

Go out to a show. Go on vacation. Visit with friends. Do something for you. Make sure the kids are well set up. Don't forget about the spouse and the pets. I am not sure why I put their spouse and their pets in the same sentence. I remind the patients they will be stuck at home after their surgery, so they should prepare whatever they need before surgery. Starting before surgery makes a big difference.

I recently spoke with Molly Sugarman, the clinical director of the Patient Empowerment Program at Aesthetics Plastic Surgery in Great Neck, New York.[35] She suggested I check out the information on breastreconstruction.org. I want to direct you to the section on the site regarding TRAM Flap reconstruction. The concepts included are extremely insightful and can be applied to many of the reconstruction procedures.

Breastreconstruction.org was created as a comprehensive resource to help women make informed choices about breast reconstruction. On the site's medical board is Dr. Ron Israeli. He has taken great care of many of my patients and I have had the fortune to observe him while performing these procedures. He and his partners do great work. Take a look for yourself.[36]

Rachel White

It's coming to the first anniversary of my first surgery of my prophylactic double mastectomy, and it's been a journey for all eight of us family members who have the BRCA1 gene. All is well. I think, as a family, we are managing. We are forever getting our boobs out and comparing. Every time I see my aunty we find a private room and compare boobs. I have had these babies out on show more than I would have ever believed it. I have never shown my boobs to anyone before this;

it's quite comical, but I am chuffed to bits with them. It's not all bad times; you can have fun after mastectomy.

Lisa Reibman

Dear Dr. Herman and Dr. Korn,

I'm truly blessed. I was one of the lucky women who happens to have two of the best doctors.

My lifesaving experience started when Dr. Herman tested me for the BRCA mutation. When I received the news I was BRCA1 positive, I didn't know how my life was about to change. Dr. Herman called me and my husband into his office. He explained and educated me on the risks, my options, and the surgeries. He performed my oophorectomy and has become, as well as my doctor, my friend.

I consider myself twice blessed, because I was to experience another life changing surgery, my mastectomy. Dr. Peter Korn reconstructed my breasts after my double mastectomy. This time, I was given options, including one I'd never heard about. I had a TUG flap reconstruction, a twelve-hour surgery. I could not have asked to be placed in more competent hands. Dr. Korn is truly one of a kind; I like to refer to him as an "Artist" with extreme knowledge of his field.

Thank you, Dr. Herman and Dr. Korn, for taking my parts and making me whole!

P.S. *In addition to Dr. Korn's medical knowledge, my follow up was three more minor surgeries, an incredible bedside manner, never a question too small. He checked me every week for months, until I was* *perfect. Now that's a doctor!*

DeAnna Howe Rice
From Her Book, January 2, 1995

Well, it was midnight the eve of my surgery. I hadn't been afraid of the surgery until then. I was afraid of dying. I trust Dr. Love, but I was still scared. If I died, Phillip, my son, would never remember me or know how much joy he brought into our lives.

Jordan would barely remember me. Raquel would remember me, but I'm sure it would grow faint. What would they remember about me? The yelling, the rushing around. Would they remember how much I loved them? Hopefully. All I have ever wanted was a family to love and care for. I do love them very much. Looking at them and watching them grow up is such a joy. I need to slow down and make sure they know how much joy they bring to me.

This is silly. I just couldn't shake this feeling. I knew I wasn't going to die. Okay, I needed to be more patient and reprioritize my life. Patience was what I planned to work on. They needed to know I always love them. I was really worried about Raquel. I rely on her too much. She is so helpful and she helped me with everything. We were in for a rough year, and I didn't want her to slip into a role in which she could not be a little girl any more.

If I could have one wish for my family it would be for my kids to love and cherish one another, to realize how special it is to have a family. I want a big, happy, and loving family. That is my dream.

Voices from the Crowd

Lulu Luke
Am I Nuts?

At first I thought I would definitely have a bilateral mastectomy and reconstruction, but over the last nine months, I have gone back and forth over the decision. Some people think I'm nuts to consider having such drastic surgery, and others think I'm mental if I don't choose surgery. I have gone 'round and 'round in circles, and I'm still undecided about mastectomy.

Pat DiRico

My ovaries and fallopian tubes were removed in January 2009. In May of 2009, I decided to see both the breast surgeon and plastic surgeon for opinions and options about my breasts. I decided to have a prophylactic double mastectomy with reconstruction in July. The last part of the reconstruction was May 2010. I am amazed at how wonderful and "real" my breasts look!

Raechel Maki
C-Cup

I could potentially end up with C-cup-sized breasts that my insurance paid for! My reconstruction has the benefit of being done without the setback of chemo or radiation. I have always had small breasts, and the thought of being able to wear a strapless dress or top without loads of tape and padded bras after my reconstruction is so exciting. I had thought of breast augmentation in the past, but never could justify spending the money on it.

Suhir Jibreen

Lovely Ladies and Gents, I found out a little over a year ago, I am a carrier of the BRCA1 gene. My cousin had breast cancer twice and eventually a double mastectomy. She has it. My mum's got it, although, thank God, she is healthy at sixty-two. Two of my aunts have it and an uncle. It's been passed to most of my cousins--boys and girls. I am currently researching and looking into the next step, but for me I don't feel I have a choice. A double mastectomy is the only way. But that's just me.

Nipples or Not?

Teri

I went with my husband to a FORCE meeting of BRCA positives. Toward the end of the session, the blinds were drawn, the doors were closed, and the men were sent out of the room. There were only two men: a BRCA1-positive man, and my husband, Travis. The women did a show and tell.

Seeing pictures of the reconstruction surgery over the internet is one thing, but to be able to see it up close and personal is another. I was amazed at how good they all looked. I'm not going to lie; they weren't perfect. They had scars, and no nipples or nipples tattooed on. One woman was in the process of having nipples recreated using excess skin and tattoos. Overall, they looked great. Under their shirts, no one would ever guess they'd had bilateral mastectomies. They could even wear bikinis and no one would know the difference.

Marcey L.

Hi all, I am scheduled for my BPM and, all of a sudden, I'm wondering about nipple sparing. Is this an option for BRCA1-positive women? At first, I didn't want to take any chances, but now I am unsure. Any thoughts or information? I read cancer originating in the nipple has never been documented, although it can travel there from other places.

Note from Teri: *It's not a true statement that cancer* never *originates in the nipples. It is, however, a rare occurrence, and if it does happen it is usually a result of having Paget's Disease.*[37]

Krystin Tate

Teri, which did you choose, and why did you make the choice you did? What information did your surgeons share with you regarding each option? *(Regarding nipple sparing.)*

Teri

All the way up until about two weeks before my PBM, I was sure I was going to have them take my nipples. Well, I changed my mind. I find it weird how different doctors have different statistics for the same thing. Anyway, my breast surgeon at the Center for Restorative Breast Surgery in New Orleans told me I was a good candidate for nipple sparing. She also told me it's rare for breast cancer to form in the nipple. Unless you have Paget's disease, it doesn't usually happen. My breast surgeon also told me I could keep them for a trial period, and if I didn't feel comfortable by the time my stage two revision surgery came around, they could remove them then.

For many breast surgeons, nipple sparing is a relatively new idea. As long as they are sure to get as much breast tissue out of there as possible, I don't see how it's any different than skin sparing, which I also had. It's a personal choice, but I do feel there is a lot of conflicting information out there that makes it a little harder for us to make informed choices.

Dr. Herman

Initially, my reaction to the concept of nipple sparring was absolutely, positively no; no how, no way. If the patient was going ahead with a mastectomy and reconstruction, she should do it right. Don't do a half-assed job. The nipples have to go. Why would any woman choose to reduce her risk, and then voluntarily leave some breast tissue behind, increasing the chance to get breast cancer? Over time, my attitude changed.

My patients would bring up the topic often. They wanted my opinion. I felt a strong obligation to research it, because I couldn't reconcile my opposition to it versus the surgeons' willingness to allow it. After reviewing the literature--I must have reviewed twenty to twenty-five papers--I concluded that, although I may not choose a nipple-sparing mastectomy for my own family, it certainly is not as objectionable as I once believed.

Voices from the Crowd

Cindi
Unsure of What's Best

I've been hesitant from the beginning about keeping my nipples or doing any sort of nipple reconstruction. There are so many issues with nipple reconstruction and nipple sparing I've heard that I just don't think it's worth it, for me. My DIEP will require a few stages, at least three trips to New Orleans-- one for the initial surgery, and then another for the revision surgery, and again for tattooing—if I go that route. I was told I could have them do the nipple sparing during the first stage, and if I decide I don't want to keep them or don't like them then, they can remove them during my revision surgery.

The purpose of nipple sparing is mostly for aesthetics. They don't typically respond to cold/touch since most of the inside has been scraped out and replaced with other fat. I'm still a little bit on the fence as far as nipples go, but I'm more than ninety percent sure I don't want to keep them. It's nice to know I can try it, and then if I change my mind, they can remove them during my second stage.

Angela
Why Doctors Say Nipples Off

From what I understand, a lot of breast cancers originate in the milk ducts of the breast. The nipple is like the meeting point for all of these ducts, so milk can be excreted from the mother to the baby. The nipple naturally has these ducts in its tissue that can harbor a five-percent cancer risk, even after having a PBM. That's why most surgeons don't want their patients to do the nipple-sparing procedures. That's what I understood, and that's what my doctor told me.

Some people might say it's just as risky having a skin-sparing mastectomy, because it is still breast tissue, but I guess the main thing are those milk ducts. Those are what can hide cancer in them.

Note from Teri: *Some of the above statements have partial misinformation and that's part of the reason we are writing this book.*

Patients are being given incorrect information and basing very important, life-altering, permanent decisions off of that.

Sharon Jack
Nipples Off

I chose not to keep mine, two years ago. I was advised by my surgeon there was a small risk, although my daughter had her PBM at the same hospital last year, and she was advised the risk was so minimal that she kept her nipples. It was my personal decision, and I am very happy with the outcome. I have had nipple reconstruction, but have yet to have them tattooed. There is a long waiting list to have them done on the NHS here in the UK.[38]

Anna
Keeping My Nipples

I am keeping my nipples. For a long while, my surgeon was planning to remove them, but just last appointment he changed his mind. He was going to leave them because he had been to a few conferences since that had said the extra benefit from removing my nipples was incredibly small. They are going to take cells from behind my nipple during the surgery and, if there is anything suspicious there at all, then they will go back and remove them.

Jamie Lou

When I originally had a nipple-sparing mastectomy, there was not as much info about how much tissue to leave in order for them to thrive, so scoop-outs went a bit too shallow for a lot of us. Surgeons were then only starting to figure out that, if they leave some of the tissue underneath the areola area, they got better vascular health.

Lee
Nipple Grafts

I guess I had the skin-sparing one. I've had one surgery to remove and replace and graft my nipples back on. I'm happy with the results. I had some healing issues where they grafted my nipples--one just didn't want to heal--but it did eventually. One nipple still pokes out, while the other won't, it's relatively flat I think due to the healing issue, maybe it scarred to much or something. I will look into other options in the future to see if the nipple can be fixed or altered. I haven't yet, because two months after surgery, I moved to another state and haven't been able to continue seeing my surgeon. Like I said, I'm happy. I can't feel anything around my nipples or near the center parts of my breasts, just the outer edges. Just thought I'd give you my experience.

Note from Teri: *It's scary that some patients have had surgeries already and aren't even aware of exactly what they've had done. Nipple grafting is not the same thing as nipple sparing. Doctors must take the time to properly explain to their patient what procedure is being performed on their patients.*

Helen Smith
I Did Nipple Sparing

My docs said they would scrape so much away, all they would leave behind was some skin. She also talked about Paget's being rare and that she did quite a few of these when she was working in Los Angeles. In good ol' conservative Ohio, I was among the first to do the nipple sparing. I was going to have them get rid of them until my doctor talked me out of it. I still have mixed feelings, since the right one had so much trouble, but at the end of the day, it did help me feel more at ease.

Helen Smith
My Nipples Aren't Symmetrical

It's tough. I am at a point where they are not symmetrical; I go in Friday for my stage two. I have asked my plastic surgeon to at least try to make them look like they are closer than they are. I don't expect them to be perfect, but I would like them to at least look a little more in line. They are googly-eyed right now.

Karin Aguirre
Didn't Spare the Nipple

I did the non-nipple-sparing surgery. My surgeon actually made the choice! He said five percent of breast cancer is hidden behind the nipple. I do, however, miss my nipples!

Note from Teri: *That seems like an odd fact to me, and one I've never heard. Doctors need to realize that we, as their patients, often completely rely on their judgment. Knowing that body parts are being removed or not, based on information (or MIS-information, as the case may be) that comes from you, is an important aspect of being a doctor. Please don't do your patients a disservice by stating opinions as facts or not being current on relevant medical information.*

Laura Dart
I Did Nipples Off

I was told that the nipple is still breast tissue, and the reason for doing PBM is to cut my chances as much as possible. I had them removed. I miss them but going for some new ones.

Lisa Edwards
Nipples Off

I chose to remove them as well, because I figured, if I were going to be aggressive, I might as well take everything.

Kay Doran
My Dr. Decided Nipples Off

I never even got the choice. My surgeon pointblank refused! I don't really miss them, but I'm still having them done later.

Sina
I Did Nipples Off

My choice was made for me. I miss my nipples.

Teri
November 10, 2009: Nipple Research

I still don't think I'm going to have nipples reconstructed. From what I understand, nipple reconstruction still hasn't been perfected. They tend to fade out and flatten out over time. I might just have some 3D nipple tattoos done. I'm just not real sure yet. I need to do more nipple research. Not a sentence I ever really imagined myself typing.

Update: *In the end, I did decide to do nipple sparing.*

Sharon Jack
Nipples Are Breast Tissue

I was told that nipple is still breast tissue and the reason for doing PBM is to cut my chances as much as possible. It was my choice to have them removed. In my case (I had a skin-sparing DIEP reconstruction), the surgeon removed the breast tissue and refilled my breasts with abdominal tissue via a circular area cutout where my nipple had been. They used skin from my stomach to cover the two areas. This means the only scars I have on my breast are the circles on each breast. The skin inside this area can be tweaked to make new nipples and the scars incorporated into the tattooing for the areola.

Debbie C.
Nipples Off

I did not keep my nipples, because both my mom and sister had ductal cancers and my breast surgeon said that it would be a risk if I kept them. She left the decision up to me, and I did not want to chance it. I will be getting redesigned nipples and tattooing.

Lisa Edwards

A family history of DCIS would be a good reason to hesitate to keep them. It all comes down, once again, to personal decision and a doctor who is willing to follow it.

Heather

My doctor said it was my decision but did not recommend keeping the nipples, so I took them off. I wanted to offer one piece of advice to anyone removing nipples: take before pictures. I did not take any pictures at all and now am really regretting it. I know some people are very into documenting the entire process. I appreciate that. I felt a little weird about taking the pictures, which is funny because it's not like I am a modest person. It just felt strange to me to take clinical pictures of my breasts. Now I am nearing my exchange surgery and making decisions about the nipple tattoos. I just really wish I had pictures to show to the tattoo artist. I am very concerned about getting a bad tattoo.

Mary B.

So when it came time to consider nipple reconstruction, the possibility of 3D tattoos rather than skin grafts was a consideration. At first, I really thought that I would be doing a disservice to any future partner if I failed to get real nipples, even though the grafts would never be quite the same as the real things. But after discussing the pros and cons with friends and family (is that love or what?) and discussing options with my plastic surgeon, I decided it was way more worth it to me to never have to wear a bra again than to have nipples permanently poking out!

Post-Op Prophylactic Bilateral Mastectomy & Reconstruction

Susan Genicoff
Three Days Ago, After Sixteen Hours of Surgery

Sixteen hours of surgery ago, I was wheeled into the recovery room with perky breasts and a one-percent chance of breast cancer. At the time, I didn't feel anything but miserable. Three days later, in my own bed, I feel overwhelmingly empowered by what I had done.

I was scared to death at the diagnosis of BRCA1 positive. I gathered courage in the knowledge I could control and conquer my risk of breast and ovarian cancer. I never once waivered in my decision to do prophylactic surgery, neither am I sorry today.

As Dr. Herman said, "Those who find out they are BRCA positive become big advocates. They learn to yell to the world around them, 'Get tested!'" That is what I am now doing. I have helped to save my life, and as John Wayne might have said, I have saddled up for the rest of my ride as I spread my message and help others like me save their lives, too.

Side note from Teri: *While reading Susan's comment I could totally visualize Dr. Herman saying just that! He's absolutely right!*

Tracey Beinstock
I Had a Preventative Double Mastectomy Six Days Ago

Please don't read my story and feel bad for me. I want you to feel how I feel: *lucky and empowered*. My cancer story began when I was fifteen. My beautiful young mother was diagnosed with breast cancer at the ripe old age of thirty-eight. I was scared and embarrassed. My mom did what she had to do, surgery, and then she went on with her life.

Unfortunately, six and a half years later, my mom was diagnosed with ovarian cancer. My vibrant, young mother succumbed to her illness three short years later. She was only forty-eight. So that's how my cancer story starts.

Now let's talk about how it ends, how I made it end. It's been over eighteen years since my mom passed away. Over those years, many more family members were diagnosed with cancer. My dad, just fifty-nine, pancreatic cancer. He fought hard but passed away at sixty-two. My maternal aunt, breast cancer. She, too, fought hard but passed away almost five years after she was diagnosed. One paternal aunt, breast cancer. Another one, ovarian cancer. A paternal uncle now with prostate cancer. I am glad to say that the three of them are doing great and are well.

Tracey's Family Red Flags

Mother	breast cancer
Mother	ovarian cancer
Maternal aunt	ovarian cancer
Father	pancreatic cancer
Paternal aunt	breast cancer
Cousin	breast cancer
Ethnic Background	Ashkenazi Jewish

In 2005, I finally decided to be tested. Of course, I wasn't surprised when my blood test revealed a mutation in the BRCA1 gene. At least now I know why so many family members were getting sick.

The first part of my decision was easy. I had a wonderful husband, thirteen-year-old twin sons, and a ten-month-old daughter. I was lucky! And empowered!

I knew what I had to do. I immediately had a preventative oophorectomy and cut my chances of ovarian cancer almost down to zero percent. Not to zero but almost. However, the next part of my decision wasn't as easy.

I started going to a breast surgeon in 2006. Every four months, I would see her for a clinical exam. Once a year, I would have a mammogram and sonogram, and six months later an MRI. With each test, I prayed, *Please don't let this be the one that finds breast cancer.*

I was lucky. All of my exams, mammos, sonos, and MRIs were normal.

Do I just keep waiting for the inevitable to happen? This past summer, my forty-three-year-old cousin, who had just buried her mom four months earlier, was diagnosed with breast cancer. Now I knew what I had to do!

This is what you need to know: I had a preventative, double mastectomy and breast reconstruction six days ago. I am home from the hospital for three days now. I am tired and uncomfortable. My family has been amazing. My husband has been taking incredible care of me as have my three kids. So how do I feel now? I feel lucky, empowered, and fortunate!

Dr. Herman

Thank you so much for your letter. I have personally learned so much from you and your family over the years. I think it is important to highlight your knowledge and reaction as a fifteen year old. We practitioners must always be cognizant of the children and have ready resources for the entire family.

- *For many patients, it is no surprise when the BRCA test is positive.*
- *A risk-reducing bilateral salpingo-oophorectomy reduces the chance of ovarian cancer close to zero but not to zero. Hence the "risk-reducing."*
- *Many women feel lucky, empowered, and fortunate after a positive BRCA test, because it provides an answer to often long-sought, unanswered questions.*
- *Young children are aware when their parents have medical problems.*

When I began testing my patients, years ago, I didn't know there were so many reconstruction options. I liked the information Teri posted on her blog. I am sure there are a few practitioners who would benefit from this information.

As such, Teri goes over the different reconstruction surgeries for us.

Teri

Just so everyone knows, this topic could be an entire book in itself and in fact is a book: *The Breast Reconstruction Guidebook*, by Kathy Stelagio, which was the first BRCA book I read after learning of my own BRCA1 mutation.[39]

With that said, there are two basic groups of reconstructions: implants and tissue flaps. Implant types include saline, silicone, or gel placed after the breast tissue is removed. Implant procedures include direct to implant and expander to implant. When the implant is placed at the time of the mastectomy, the procedure is the direct to implant. When the implant is placed later on, giving the chance for expanders to stretch the skin so the proper size implant can be placed, it is known as the expander implant procedure.

In a flap procedure, tissue, including sometimes muscle and fat, is repositioned from an area of the body, refashioning them under the skin of the chest to form breast mounds. Commonly performed flaps include the *lattisimus dorsi* flap, the S-GAP, TRAM flap, DIEP flap, and hip flap.

Reconstruction can also include areola reconstruction and nipple and areola tattoos, or skin sparing and nipple sparing. Different plastic surgeons have different specialties, and doctors should be researched before settling on one.

A list of items helpful to women after surgery (and best to know about prior to surgery):

- *Diaper pins to pin the drains to your clothes, or better yet, a drain pouch*
- *Shirts that button or zip down the front*
- *A recliner chair to rest in, or lots of pillows to sleep in a propped up position*
- *Lots of baby wipes for those in-between shower days (FYI: the process of showering after a mastectomy is exhausting)*
- *A lap tray for meals*
- *Friends to drop off home-cooked meals or a stock of pre-made*

food in our freezer (FYI: Most women who have the PBM go through the same sort of "nesting mode" that a pregnant woman goes through)

- *Throat lozenges and Chapstick (waiting for them, in the recovery room!)*

Dr. Herman
About Rachel H.'s: "Losing the Boobs"

One of my favorite blogs is "Losing the Boobs." Rachel H. documents her recovery from her risk-reducing mastectomy with expander to implant reconstruction. There are so many great things about this blog. I like her personal lists of can and can't dos so much I asked if we could share them.

If you aren't familiar, post-mastectomy reconstruction with a tissue expander to implant involves a number of different stages. A tissue expander is a temporary device that is placed under the chest wall deep to the pectoralis major muscle. The purpose of the expander is to help the wall stretch over time and thus create a pocket. In the weeks following the initial surgery, the patient returns to the surgeon's office and has the expanders filled with saline (most patients will simply refer to this as "fills"). When the pocket is the correct size the implant is placed inside, during the exchange surgery.

Rachel H.
From Her Blog: "Losing the Boobs"

Things I Could Do Immediately after Surgery:

- *Get in and out of bed*

- *Go to the bathroom on my own*
- *Wipe my own a$$ (thank you, dear God!)*
- *Touch my head*

Things I Could Not Do after Surgery:

- *Put on a button/zipper sweater*
- *Lift anything more than a glass of water or wad of toilet paper*
- *Sleep on my side or stomach*

Below is a quick emergency list for your patients. **Call your doctor ASAP if you have:**

- *Difficulty breathing (possible fluid in lungs or pulmonary embolism)*
- *A fever greater than 101° (that could be a sign of infection)*
- *Nausea and vomiting that is not getting better, dizziness and/or weakness that is excessive*
- *Pain that isn't improved with medication*
- *Bright red skin that is hot to the touch (that's a sign of infection)*
- *Heavy bleeding or seepage through the incisions*
- *One breast shape very different from the other*

Possible sign of necrosis or hematoma:

- *Drains that have stopped draining*
- *Pain in the calf (sign of a DVT, deep vein thrombosis, or simply put, blood clot)*

At two to ten days post-op, a few things the plastic surgeon might tell your patients:

- *Your patient may take prescription medications and muscle* relaxants as needed; when able, switch to Tylenol

- *Your patient may shower starting two days after her surgery. The water should not be too hot and she should avoid putting anything on the incisions like soap, moisturizers, and creams.*
- *Your patient may receive clearance to begin driving at approximately one week after surgery.*
- *Your patient may return to work as soon as two weeks after surgery (four weeks would be the normal time though).*
- *Your patient must wear a support bra (unless specifically told otherwise by her doctor).*
- *Your patient must walk–walk, walk, walk! Patients who walk after surgery heal quicker. Those who lay in the bed get sick. This is a good general rule.*
- *Your patient must eat a healthy diet. No smoking and no alcohol.*

Twelve Days Post-Operative

Things I Could Do:

- *Comb, wash, dry, and style my hair including blow-drying, straightening, or putting it up in a ponytail*
- *Open and close my windows*
- *Sleep on my sides (I struggled to find that sweet spot of comfortableness)*
- *Light chores such as cooking, cleaning the litter box, dishes, disinfecting bathroom*

Things I Couldn't Do:

- *Open heavy doors*
- *Laundry*
- *Vacuuming*
- *Driving*

Two to four weeks post-operative, a few things the plastic surgeon might tell your patients:

- *Your patient may put moisturizer, creams, and/or oils on the scars once the scabs are gone. Do not expose them to the sun.*
- *Your patient must wear a support bra. No underwires.*
- *Your patient may try scar treatments like Mederma.*
- *Your patient may begin to exercise.*
- *Your patient may lift up to two pounds. Go slowly. No swinging. No bouncing. No twisting. Nothing above her head!*

Six and One-half Weeks Post-Operative:

Things I Could Do:

- *Swim (I went swimming in the river. I could dog paddle a bit but could not do the breast stroke yet. In the deep waters, I would still be in trouble if I had to swim to save my life).*
- *Sleep on my stomach. Yes! I can sleep comfortably on my stomach with expanders. I just have a lot of blankets stuffed under my chest area for padding. I am a stomach sleeper so now I have been getting a better nights rest.*
- *Wear a two-piece bikini*
- *Drive*
- *Go the whole day without a nap*
- *Work! I do a lot of childcare and am able to do all of my regular duties*
- *Lift, I am able to lift three year olds and also a case of water bottles without any pain or difficulty.*

Three Months Post-Operative:

Things I Could Do:

- *Swim (I can probably tread water for about five minutes, do*

the breast stroke, and back stroke).
- *Dive off a raft (and still lose my bottoms!)*
- *Jump off a raft to try and "touch bottom" of the lake*
- *Run*
- *Drive a standard (stick shift) transmission*
- *French braid my hair in two braids like the Dutch girl I am*

Three Months Post-Operative:

Things I Couldn't Do:

- *Chin ups*
- *Wear a bra for more than a couple of hours (it gets too uncomfortable)*
- *Sleep on my stomach, since my last expansion. I am too large to sleep comfortably on my stomach. I still get a good night's rest though by sleeping on my sides.*
- *Feel confident with a man with my shirt off in an intimate situation. Yeesh! I know this will come in time as the scars fade and the final surgery is done, but what a mood breaker. I refused for them to be touched. They feel so freakish. I am sure he would, and was fine with it, but I was just so damned self-conscious and that didn't make for a very enjoyable experience. Lights off... 'nuff said.*

After filling-up the expanders I could:

- *Swim, although not as strongly as last "can do" list, I've lost a bit of my strength.*
- *Pick up children, although it was difficult after the last fill for the first week and a half.*
- *I can still sleep on my sides, though it is starting to get a little bit uncomfortable with the increase in size.*

After filling-up the expanders I couldn't:

- *Sleep on my stomach. I tried this morning but it was completely uncomfortable and unnatural.*
- *Hug very hard. My chest is getting really tight, and it is uncomfortable to have that much pressure on my chest.*
- *I can't get completely cozy with the little kids I babysit when cuddling with them. I have to be very careful that they don't jump on me when they are excited. They are so cute! Even though they are so young, they know how to be respectful and understand that they need to be careful with me.*
- *Wear tight clothing. It feels so restricting and causes my skin to ache and feel an itchy kind of pain. This means I don't wear bras any more, and it also means I have grown out of most of my tops; thus I need to go shopping.*

Karen Malkin-Lazarovitz

Karen is well known for coining the term "Operation Squishy Boob" when referring to her exchange surgery.

Things some patients don't like about their surgery:

- *Your patient might not like the way her new breasts look (size, shape, lack of symmetry, etc.)*
- *Your patient might not like the way her scars look.*
- *Your patient might not like the way her breasts feel.*
- *Your patient might not like the loss of sensation. Over time, some sensation might return. Maybe.*
- *Your patient might have problems (lack of sensation, nerve issues) at the donor site for those who had a flap procedure.*
- *Your patient will probably become impatient, and feel as if their recovery is taking too long.*
- *Your patient probably will hate the fatigue.*
- *Your patient might require a revision surgery/stage two*

(this is a common occurrence, so it would be great to fore-warn your patients of this possibility prior to their first surgery). While it's common to need revisions, it's still dis-couraging for your patient to learn she will need one.

Cynthia Jeanne Kimball

I'm glad I had my double mastectomy reconstructive surgery. If I had to make the same decision over again today, I would do the exact same thing. There really wasn't a worst part of having a mastectomy for me. Sure, if I could have kept my natural-born breasts, that would have been ideal. To me, that wasn't an option, even though it was an option. Yes, basically it was my choice, but that choice came with a strong recom-mendation from my doctors.

To me, having a double mastectomy (with latissimus dorsi re-construction) surgery was a no brainer. The boobs had to go or eventually I might.

I remember clearly the breast surgeon asking me, "Are you sure you want to do this?"

"Of course."

"Your new breasts won't feel the same as the ones you have now."

"I've heard. But it's okay. I'm ready."

"You're sure."

"One-hundred percent."

He proceeded to tell me what my reconstructed breasts would be like, as did my plastic surgeon. I liked how my sister's reconstructed breasts turned out after her double mastectomy. I looked at before and after pictures of other patients while at my plastic surgeon's office. I visualized what my new breasts would look like. I recited positive affirmations to help prepare for this shift.

To me, the worst part would have been not making a decision. You know, should I go forward with a double mastectomy or not?

Voices from the Crowd

Raechel Maki
Nipple-Sparing Mastectomy

On September 23, 2010, at the age of thirty, I became my surgeon's fifth nipple and skin-sparing prophylactic bilateral mastectomy patient. My plastic surgeon placed tissue expanders under the muscle using Alloderm.[40]

I had a little problem with a hematoma post-op, but with a second surgery and revision, things are turning out nicely. I am on my way to recovery. Ultimately, I think I will be very happy with the results. I will have silicone implants placed after the expansion process is finished. I also don't have to feel like a ticking time bomb any more.

Karen Malkin-Lazarovitz
Family Stupidity

I have had family members tell me that I didn't need to do the surgeries and that I'm making too much of it. I even had a family member tell me it's all right that I'm in pain from the surgery, because I chose this. I guess getting cancer would be easier for them to understand. I understand stupidity from people who don't know about BRCA, but to have such insensitivity. It makes me sick. I have learned not to deal with those toxic types of people. I did what I did for my kids, my husband, and for myself. Screw everyone else who has a stupid opinion.

Sharon Osier Stanley
It Was Hard

My reconstruction will finally be done in two weeks. That is why I feel it is important to stand up and say I did this. It was really hard, and it still is hard at times. But I had to do it to save my life. I always knew I had a calling in life. Peace, love, and humanism are what I thought was my calling. The last thing I ever expected was to become a breast cancer advocate. But as John Lennon said, "Life is what happens when you're busy making other plans."[41]

Jenny D.
Waiting to Happen

My self-breast exams went from monthly, to weekly, to daily. I chose to remove my left breast. Some may call it "healthy or normal tissue," but to me it was a cancer feast waiting to happen.

P.S. *All of the doctors wanted me to remove it.*

Victoria Dockery
I'm BRCA Positive

Found out this past May. I just had my prophylactic bilateral mastectomy done four weeks ago, and I'm so happy I did it. But I have had friends and family who don't understand why we do this to our bodies. My sister is going in for her PBM. We have each other's back. My cousin had her mastectomy last week. She's only thirty. I'm thirty-six; my sister is thirty-two. We don't want cancer. Some people don't understand what it's like to be BRCA positive. That little piece of paper changes everything.

Raechel Maki

I have gotten over any form of shyness about private parts I ever had. Seriously, I could take off all my clothes in the middle of Times Square and not blink an eye.

Things Everyone Should Know About Hereditary Breast & Ovarian Cancer Syndrome

Hereditary breast and ovarian cancer syndrome (HBOC) is an inherited disorder that multiplies the risk of getting breast and/or ovarian cancer. Most cases of HBOC can be detected by testing for gene mutations known as BRCA1 and BRCA2. Genetic testing is performed from a blood or saliva sample.

BRCA mutations might explain why a patient has breast and/or ovarian cancer and might help identify additional family members with the syndrome. BRCA mutations could be inherited from one's father or mother. When a person tests positive, his or her siblings and children have a fifty-percent chance of having the mutation, too. For that reason, it's crucial to look at family history on both the maternal and paternal side of the family.

HBOC is more common in some ethnic groups, like the Ashkenazi Jews. Among Ashkenazi Jews, the chance of having a mutation is one in forty. That's about ten times higher than the general population. However, the BRCA mutation is not limited to those of Ashkenazi Jewish ancestry.[42]

Remember, BRCA testing is a risk-evaluation tool. It helps the physician give more accurate advice to patients and helps patients make better informed medical decisions.

Testing positive does not mean one will develop breast cancer, just as testing negative doesn't mean one won't.

Men can get breast cancer, too. Over two thousand per year in the US do. BRCA2 mutations increase the risk of breast cancer and prostate cancer in men.[43]

Genetic mutations cannot skip a generation. If your mother has a BRCA mutation and you don't, your daughter cannot inherit it from your side of the family.

Today, with mammography, breast MRI, ultrasound, medication and risk-reducing surgeries, people who are BRCA positive can lower their risk for cancer. Doctors can't totally nullify the risk, but it can be reduced by more than ninety-plus percent. BRCA testing saves lives.

One of the biggest problems is that the majority of people who have a BRCA mutation don't even know it. Awareness is critical to saving lives.

If your patient has breast or ovarian cancer in her family, talk with her. Don't miss the opportunity! It just might save her life! If you know someone with breast and/or ovarian cancer tell her about HBOC and BRCA.

SECTION TWO

Stories & Letters

LISA'S STORY

A Family Intervention

Teri
Question for Dr. Herman

You deliver babies, you operate, you see patients in your office, you are involved in research, you teach. How do you have the time to travel all over the U.S. to get the word out about BRCA mutations?

Dr. Herman

Well, the truth is, I don't have the time. That's for sure. I do feel it is so important to make time. So I do. I do it for the patients, the people I have met, the people I have connected with through Facebook and blogs and their families. Recently, I saw two patients I delivered over fifteen years ago, long before I knew about BRCA genes, who only now did I discover are BRCA positive. Their story pushes me to make the time.

Since 2006, I have received many BRCA-related letters. I have kept every one. Each tells of a personal story. Each one has its own important message. There are two that really stand out.

When I feel like giving up, when I am post call, heading to the airport to go lecture, leaving my family, these two letters remind me of why I keep pushing myself. I keep them on my laptop, and I carry a few copies around with me to share when I teach. I would say I am very proud of them.

Here is the first, Lisa's Story, and later on, please don't miss reading Tiffany's.

Lisa
I Teach about BRCA for a Living

Dear Dr. Herman, I wanted to share with you how you have personally impacted my life and the lives of several of my family members. Last month, while we drove all over North Carolina teaching healthcare professionals about hereditary cancer syndromes, we chatted about my coworker's and my family history.

I lost my mom; a maternal aunt, Anne; her daughter (my cousin), Samantha; all to ovarian cancer. I have only one cancer survivor relative left, my cousin, Barbara (Anne's daughter), who was diagnosed with breast cancer at age forty-two.

Lisa's Mother	*ovarian cancer*
Maternal aunt (Anne)	*ovarian cancer*
Cousin (Anne's daughter, Samantha)	*ovarian cancer*
Cousin (Anne's daughter, Barbara)	*breast cancer (42)*

When I first started educating about BRCA, I suggested to Barbara she be tested, but this fell on deaf ears. She didn't pursue it.

Dr. Herman, you reminded me that I talk to doctors every day about hereditary cancer syndromes, and I have an entire family who could possibly benefit from knowing our BRCA status, not to mention how I would feel if another of my relatives were to be diagnosed with breast or ovarian cancer, then I were to later find out that indeed there was a BRCA mutation in the family. Your words really haunted me.

A week and a half after your visit, I decided it was time for a "family intervention." On Sunday afternoon, I gathered eight cousins and my aunt around my kitchen table. I had prepared a five-generation pedigree chart and reviewed our family's cancer history as well as the risk assessment booklet. My cousin, Barbara, the breast cancer survivor, agreed that she had to be tested.

During our intervention, I discovered that eleven years after Barbara's mastectomy, she was diagnosed with breast cancer in the other breast! I just about fell out of my chair. I was in college at the time of her second diagnosis, and I never knew it. Fortunately, the second cancer was discovered early and was successfully treated with lumpectomy and radiation. I guess, by now, you know where I am going with my story.

Two days after our family meeting, I joined Barbara for her blood draw. A week later, we discovered she tested positive for the BRCA1 mutation! Several days later, my Aunt Sally went in for testing, too. She, too, tested positive for the BRCA1 mutation. Next, her daughter (my cousin) Kathy, who was thirty-eight and who had not ever even had a mammogram, went in for testing. A well-respected breast surgeon in town, (who attended one of your presentations), was the physician who met with several of my family members. He's now managing our entire family.

During Kathy's clinical breast exam, the doctor felt something suspicious. He sent her for a mammogram, but the mammogram showed nothing. Given our family history, he then sent her for an ultrasound that confirmed what he had felt. An hour later, she had a breast biopsy. We were all on pins and needles waiting for the results.

It has all been very surreal. I think we all are in shock. I just received an email tonight that two more cousins are going in for testing next week.

While waiting for the biopsy results, Kathy made quite a profound comment, "What if the biopsy does find something? Think about what it could have been had I waited until I was forty for my baseline mammogram?"

We now have six more relatives who need to be tested and their results will directly impact fifty-nine more family members, all from our conversation in the car driving through the boondocks of North Carolina.

Dr. Herman, thank you, thank you, thank you. What a story we can share. We must, because there are so many more families like mine.

Congrats on all the exciting news! You are changing and saving so many lives. Your book will get the word out even more. Thank you so much for all that you do!

P.S. *It was a long weekend, but on the following Tuesday, Kathy's pathology report arrived and it was negative! She later found out she is BRCA negative.*

Teri

Just... Wow! There are so many important lessons from Lisa's story. Dr. H., what do you think is the most important message practitioners should take away from a story like Lisa's?

Dr. Herman

The take home message: It's so easy to let your patients go untested. I hear it all the time. "I told my patient about it and sent her to genetics, and she didn't go." Make it a priority to get testing done for those who should have it. Educate your patients and they will respond.

Voices from the Crowd

Gail Mankiewicz

Thank you for reminding us we have a responsibility to inform other family members about the possibility of being BRCA positive. Our silence could cost some of them their lives.

DeAnna Howe Rice

Reasons to get tested:

- *It might help your patient avoid breast cancer.*
- *It might help your patient avoid ovarian cancer.*
- *It might save your patient from chemotherapy.*
- *It might save your patient from radiation treatments.*
- *It will help you more effectively treat your patient.*

- *It will allow your patient to be here for her children.*
- *It would explain why your patient's mother died from breast or ovarian cancer.*
- *It might save your patient's sisters.*
- *It might save your patient's extended family members.*
- *It will bring your patients peace of mind.*
- *It gives her a chance to be proactive and empowered.*

Teri

It's so sad how so many have to act like a rabid pit bull to get doctors to listen to them. I can't believe the amount of women denied genetic counseling for no apparent or logical reason. So many people in the medical community need to be woken up!

Dr. Herman

Teri, I love how you put that. I read a paper in 2009 I always think about. Among women deemed at high risk of HBOC, fifty-four percent had heard of genetic testing for cancer risk, just over ten percent had discussed genetic testing for cancer risk with a health professional, fewer than five percent were advised by a health professional to be tested, and fewer than two percent actually underwent testing.

Only a small minority of women who need BRCA testing have it done. Teri, in your opinion, can you tell me why do you think so few people have been tested?

Teri

My thoughts are that this question has a multitude of mini answers. I could look to the doctors, or I could look to the patients as responsible. I personally think the responsibility falls with both.

How many times have I had to arrive at my doctor's appointment early to fill out a thick packet of paperwork? It's common practice, and in fact, sometimes it's requested, that the patient pick up the paperwork beforehand, so she has time to complete it at home. As my fingers cramp up from filling all the pages out, I sometimes can't help but feel annoyed. Is anyone even going to read any of this stuff? My experience has been that it may be glanced over during your initial consultation, but after that, it's sealed up in a tomb with inches of dust settling on top.

When I first learned the BRCA mutation ran in my family, it was the first time I could recall hearing the acronym. I knew nothing of it. I didn't grow up fearful of breast or ovarian cancer. I didn't know my family history pre-BRCA diagnosis, as I do now. I didn't know that I didn't know. I didn't know that if I went looking, I might find some scary stuff. I didn't know any of this, until someone told me about it, a family member.

Had I been a bigger advocate of my own health in my mid-thirties, surfed the net more or paid more attention to medical news going on around me, perhaps I would have known more about it. The point is, I don't live like that. I don't live looking for the next big thing that's wrong with me. I don't seek out health problems that I've never even heard of. I'd be willing to bet the average person doesn't do this either. And here is where I think a big part of the responsibility lies with the doctors.

I give you this hypothetical scenario:

Dr. Supersmart gets a new patient. He has fifteen other patients in the waiting room and more scheduled to come in at fifteen-minute intervals throughout the day. Each patient is scheduled for roughly a ten, maybe fifteen-minute exam with him. He has a wife at home always nagging him for being at the office so much and kids who are disappointed in him because he never makes it to their soccer games. It eats at the back of his mind, but he's a good doctor, and he needs to stay focused. He'll worry about all that other stuff later. And yes, he was thinking about all of that, while flipping through his new patient's family history that was so diligently filled out.

Doctors are overbooked, appointments aren't long enough, and as far as OB/GYNs are concerned (who might make up the bulk of doctors that would catch the BRCA/HBOC connection), the day doesn't start at 8:00 and end at 5:00. Far from it. They get up early, hightail it to the hospital where they make the rounds, quickly check-in on their patients, talk to the nurses who took care of their patients all night, sign things here, order prescriptions or tests there, then hoof it over to their office to start their very busy day.

Sometimes they make it to lunch by noon, other times not. You never know when a pregnant woman is going to be ready to deliver her baby (unless it's a planned cesarean section). It may happen right at the end of office hours, as Dr. Supersmart is sitting at his desk about to do what good doctors do, and read through his patients' files, and determine the best course of action. His pager goes off and he learns Mrs. Forty Weeks is on labor and delivery at the hospital with her water broken, and three other pregnant women are calling the after-hours emergency number because they just can't stand the heartburn any more, the hiccups won't go away and they hurt, or they haven't felt movement for three hours. In light of all of this, of course Dr. Supersmart doesn't have time to sit and read through files looking for potential problems. He has to attend to the immediately pressing ones.

He returns phone calls while rushing back to the hospital, makes one last call to apologize to his wife that he's going to have to miss dinner, again, and on to labor and delivery he rushes to save the day. A few hours later, he finishes up, breathes a sigh of relief while he gets in his car and heads home. Too tired from such a long day, he hits the sack, only to be jarred awake at midnight that he's needed back at the hospital. It's a vicious cycle, and with all that on Dr. Supersmart's shoulders, can this really be any more his fault than that of his patient who may or may not have a hereditary disposition to breast or ovarian cancer?

Is there a solution? Sure there is!

Here is an idea: Doctors have staff! Very capable, very competent staff! The task of looking through patients' family histories for tells of HBOC/BRCA could be given to one of the medical assistants. It could be a task expected to be taken care of every Wednesday from 9:15a.m. to 2:45p.m., or some other time that fits into the schedule best. Some people are especially good with computers and databases. Their skills could and should be utilized. Let them create a database (or purchase an existing software that does this already) that has the ability to flag problem areas/patients.

Another assistant could be in charge of data entry, and they would spend X amount of hours per day (or any downtime) inputting patient records into the database. Once per morning or once per week, a report can be run where all the people who fit the profile of a BRCA mutant gets pulled up in a list.

Set aside one day every two weeks and schedule the doctor's day for these patients only. Of course, women will still be having babies while all of this is going on, and you'll just have to roll with that, but just because something seems hard doesn't mean it's impossible.

Dr. Herman

Teri, your point is well taken. Gyns need to pay attention from the get-go and be aggressively looking when our patients come to see us. Now a lot of us have electronic medical records (EMR) and electronic health records (EHR) that can be utilized.[44]

I see a bigger problem. We doctors, ourselves, have to be knowledgeable about BRCA before we can look for it. We need to know who to look for, why it's important, what the results mean: who, what, where, why, and when.

On January 3, 2008, I gave grand rounds. I arrived a few minutes early while they were doing tumor board. Everyone was there: the gynecologist, the chemotherapy people, the radiation people, the residents, the attendings. The chief resident was presenting the case. Together, they would formulate a multi-disciplinary approach to the treatment plan. Keep in mind how many people we have involved in taking care of this patient.

When I heard the story, I took the paper. I took it off the table, and I slid it in my bag. It says: forty-eight-year-old female newly diagnosed with stage IIIC ovarian cancer.

What's going to happen to her? Sadly, she's going to die, in all likelihood. But what do I want to know as the BRCA person who was about to give grand rounds on hereditary breast and ovarian cancer?

What is her family history? Just below the middle of the page it says: mother with breast cancer and aunt with breast cancer. Listen to this. This resident who's going to graduate in six months and go out to practice medicine is standing up in front of the GYN/ONCs, the oncologists, the radiation people, the attendings, and so on. He suggested her treatment plan: chemotherapy.

It should have been chemotherapy and BRCA testing. We are taught on day one to take a proper history. He missed it because he didn't ask the proper questions. He didn't know to ask them.

- *At what age did her mother have breast cancer?*
- *Was it in one breast or both?*
- *Did the breast cancer come back again?*
- *What is her ethnic background?*
- *Who is the aunt? Is she on the maternal side or the paternal side?*
- *At what age did the aunt have breast cancer?*

So her treatment plan should have included chemotherapy and BRCA testing on behalf of her children, and her aunt, and her other aunt, and her sister, and her brother, and whoever else was in the family. Because she may have six brothers and sisters, and they might all have six kids. We have to stop letting opportunities pass us by.

So why aren't people tested for BRCA mutations? Because the chief resident didn't think about it and ask the proper questions when the opportunity arose.

Dr. Robert P.

We need to take a good history—every year—on every patient. Thank you for reminding me that BRCA mutations can come through the paternal line as well.

Gail Mankiewicz
RE: Dr. Supersmart

I think doctors need to schedule fewer appointments in order to take better care of their patients. Is this a crazy idea or what?)

Note from Teri: *Gail, that isn't a crazy idea, but it's not always possible or realistic. In the small town I'm from, there were exactly two OB/GYNs, and one was well past retirement age, just unable to retire because of too many patients and not enough doctors to see them all.*

DeAnna Howe Rice
Things I Wish You Had Told Me

- *BRCA testing was covered by my insurance*
- *There was a law that protected me from discrimination (GINA)*
- *That I didn't have to have a mastectomy if I came back positive for a BRCA mutation*
- *That there are options under the medical management tree*
- *That being BRCA positive could be a good thing in my life*
- *That I wasn't alone*
- *That I could help save lives*

Amy S.

When I went for an appointment with a genetic nurse, she tried to talk me out of getting testing. "It's highly unlikely that you'll have a positive result."

Well, she had to eat those words.

Amy Yoffe

I've wanted to get tested for years. My OB/GYN told me that my family history isn't relevant because it's on my father's side. He also told me that since my mother wasn't born Jewish, it would water down the gene. Both those things turned out to be incorrect.

Dr. Z.

I teach my staff, "We are the patient's advocates. Don't forget, we work for them."

Christine Slagmulder Kempton

I inherited it from my dad. Even though four of his female relatives had breast cancer, not one of my past three physicians suggested genetic counseling. One physician, in 1995, even suggested I didn't need to worry as much since it was on my paternal side. I had one mammography tech tell me that they only look at the maternal side for family history. I inherited my mutation from my father.

Alison
I Should Have Never Gotten Cancer

I was diagnosed with breast cancer at age sixty-two. I followed my oncologist's plan and had a lumpectomy, followed by radiation treatments. Six months later, my gynecologist suggested BRCA testing, because of my family and personal history.

I did test, and I am BRCA2 positive. I have to tell you... I'm angry. First, the oncologist should have known I was BRCA positive before she set up my treatment plan. I shouldn't have had a lumpectomy, and I shouldn't have had radiation. I should have had a mastectomy and then breast reconstruction. It was the wrong operation. Now that I had radiation, I am having a hard time finding a competent breast surgeon and plastic surgeon to take care of my comprised skin.

Now here is the worse part: I had my ovaries and fallopian tubes out and my gynecologist found early fallopian tube cancer. Maybe I will be lucky, because it was found early, no thanks to my oncologist. However, I shouldn't have gotten it in the first place. I shouldn't have needed the chemotherapy that's killing me. The truth is, I should have never had breast cancer to begin with, because someone should have figured this out years ago.

TIFFANY'S STORY

Running Scared

Tiffany Reiss

I choose this title because it was the actual act of running that led me to the right people. I was fourteen when I was told my mom was sick. I was at sleep-away camp and was told mom was in the hospital having a minor surgery. My dad didn't want me to worry. The truth was, she was undergoing a complete hysterectomy. At the age of thirty-eight, my mother, Shevi Reiss, was diagnosed with stage IV ovarian cancer. No signs, no symptoms, not a single person in the family prior to her had been sick.

How then was it possible she was so sick? At the time, I didn't really know what it all meant and always assumed she would be just fine. I knew cancer was bad, but I had hope. I mean, as a child, when you get sick, you go to the doctor, and they give you a prescription for something, you go home, a few days go by, and you get better. That was all I really knew about being sick. I learned much more about it in the coming years.

Mom wasn't just sick; she was dying. Ovarian cancer, the silent killer, was taking away my mother's most beautiful years. Cancer threatened her dreams of seeing her two daughters through all the wonderful stages of our lives. Mom fought for about three years until ovarian cancer ultimately delivered her fate. Mom died on Rosh Hashanah 1990. They say only really special chosen ones die on that day. I would have rather her not been so special. She missed my high school graduation, college graduation, my wedding, my firstborn, my second born, and the chance to be the most wonderful grandparent alive.

Now, she is missing her daughter's triumphant decisions to live beyond age thirty-eight!

I was told something about a gene test about eight years back. Every time I inquired about it to my gynecologist, I got the runaround. Either I was given a phone number to call, to no avail, or a blank stare. There was even one who told me she had no idea what I was talking about but would look into it for me. That never happened.

Time passed and I was raising two children, living on Long Island, buying my first house, and living the dream. Genetic testing wasn't the first thing on my mind. I guess I figured one day someone would know what to do. I trusted my doctors, and if they didn't know about it, well then, maybe it didn't really exist. But I have to say, always trust your gut, because deep down inside, I knew I had to pursue a bit harder. Plus, my dad kept pushing for it as well. I was stuck and didn't know where to turn. It was a challenge and struggle to get to the right place.

Raising two young children became my focus and other things took a backseat to them. I decided the least I could do was live healthier, so I started running. I had never really run before! I felt the need to run. I decided to tell everyone I was going to complete a marathon in my mother's honor.

Just in case you don't know this, when one says they are going to run a marathon, unless you break your foot, you're doing it.

So I trained. I ran into a girl named Heather at a mutual friend's child's birthday party. I had met Heather when I first moved into the neighborhood, but we didn't become friends just then. We were both admiring how dry our hands were and got on the topic of running. See, we both ran outside in the dead of winter and our hands were dry.

She asked me how much I ran, and I told her I was in training for a marathon. She said, "Me, too." And here is where the title comes in: We ran religiously together at 5a.m.

She had one rule: No talking while we run. I agreed to the no-talking rule, and the first morning, we talked the entire run through, and thus, she saved my life. Not only had our paths crossed before, but she knew the one piece of information that would change my life forever.

After hearing the story about my mom, she told me about a doctor who spoke at her friend's house about a gene test. She urged me to call him that same morning. I never even knew the name of it before that day. When I got home, I made the call to a Dr. Herman. I made an appointment to come in, and within a week, I was sitting in his office. This very passionate, kind man introduced himself to me and told me I was in the right place. We talked about my mom and her family history and found out things I never thought would be important.

For instance, my mother's paternal aunt died of breast cancer at age seventy. *Aha!* The link. My mom's dad's sister had breast cancer. But what did that prove? It proved that through my grandfather, my mom got this gene that predisposed her to breast and ovarian cancer. It also made cancer appear to have skipped a generation, because it came through my grandfather's line. So since my mom was so young and her aunt did not yet have cancer, she was the first. Correction, she was the youngest.

Tiffany's Family Red Flags

Mother	ovarian cancer
Maternal side great aunt	breast cancer
Ethnic Background	Ashkenazi Jewish Ancestry

So, Dr. Herman suggested that my sister, Lauren, and I take the test for the Ashkenazi Jewish founder mutations. He said it would help determine if a broken gene that connects breast and ovarian cancer has been passed down to us. Okay, so what next? I figured this must be some great big to-do of a test. Wrong again. "Go into the exam room and give blood."

What? Give blood? It's a simple blood test? I couldn't believe my ears. I have been searching for a test that can save my life that takes three seconds to do, and not one single doctor I met ever knew about it. I was floored, frustrated, relieved, angry, all of it. But of all the feelings I had, thankful was the most dominant! It was supposed to take two to four weeks for an answer.

I took the test May 2, 2007 and received the results on May 14, 2007. Dr. Herman informed me I was BRCA1 positive. My sister also came back positive. What we were told that meant at the time was we had an eighty-seven-percent chance of breast cancer and a forty-four-percent chance of ovarian cancer by age seventy. Age seventy. Wait a minute. I am only thirty-three, and mom was only thirty-eight.

Dr. Herman advised me to come in and discuss my options. I did so the very next day. I already knew what I had to do for me. I made the decision to have a prophylactic double mastectomy with reconstruction and a salpingo-oopherectomy.

My sister made the same decisions. It was the most empowered I had ever felt in my whole life. It was the one decision I knew was 100 percent right for me. Now, I was going to see my children through all the amazing stages of their lives. Graduations, weddings, births, and becoming a grandparent were all real possibilities.

On June 19, 2007, I underwent my first of many surgeries. I had a wonderful team. Dr. Gordon did the mastectomy (I was the last patient of his career), Dr. Leipziger did my reconstruction (beyond amazing, he put me back together) and Dr. Herman my oophorectomy (the man is a walking angel).

Marathoners Heather and Tiffany

I thank these doctors for this great BRCA news! For spreading the word and saving lives. I thank them for giving me the opportunity to make a decision that would change my life. It was truly a gift. I no longer worry that I, too, will be prey to my mother's fate. My prophylactic double mastectomy revealed an in-situ breast cancer. It was so early, but today, instead of writing this article and recovering from breast cancer, I'm writing this letter recovering from surgeries I chose to have in order to save my life. I am no longer running scared.

- *Children are aware when their parents have medical problems.*
- *BRCA mutations may appear to have skipped a generation when it passes through the paternal side.*
- *Many healthcare providers are unaware of the importance of BRCA testing.*
- *Spreading the word about BRCA and HBOC saves lives.*
- *The opportunity to make decisions and take action is empowering.*

Dr. Lyle Leipziger is the Chief of the Division of Plastic and Recon-

*structive Surgery at North Shore University Hospital (NSUH[45])
and Long Island Jewish Medical Center (LIJMC[46]) and has served in
that capacity since 1994 at LIJMC and 1999 at NSUH.*

Dr. Herman

You just read the story. Thirty-four year old Tiffany showed
up in my office and said to me, "I went to my doctor three
years in a row, and I asked for BRCA testing, because my
mother had ovarian cancer at thirty-eight and died at forty-
two. I have some breast cancer in the family also. You know
what my doctor did? She blew me off, three years in a row. I
need this done."

I said, "Fine." I explained it. I said, "Okay, let's take your
blood." And she almost fell on the floor.

"This is only a blood test? This is just a simple blood test?"

I said, "Tiffany, the blood test is simple, but everything that
goes with it is a lot more complicated."

So I took her blood, and her sister came two weeks later, and I
took her blood also. They both came back BRCA positive. One
of my "great days in medicine" was when I took out both their
tubes and ovaries on the same day. Both came back benign,
and they both elected to have mastectomies with bilateral
breast reconstruction. And that was done. What happened
next? Tiffany went on vacation to Bermuda, and she, in the
Princess Something or Other Hotel, ran into Dr. Phil. (*The* Dr.
Phil[47]). She saw him in the lobby, and told her husband, "I'm
going to go speak to him." Because you know what happens
when patients test positive? They become big advocates. If

they see somebody in a supermarket, they overhear them talking about someone who has breast cancer, they'll say, "Excuse me for being rude, but do you know that there's this test that could help save the family?"

They'll stop anybody, anywhere.

Tiffany speaks to Dr. Phil, and says, "This is my story."

He said, "This is not for my show, but my son and I, we're starting this show called The Doctors." And a month later, we were on a plane, we went to Hollywood, and I was on the show. I was on TV for a few minutes, but I'm telling you the story for another reason.

I'm telling you because they asked her a question: "Did you expect to come back positive?"

Tiffany gave the strangest answer. She said something like, "I didn't expect to come back positive, but I was hoping that I would."

Strange answer.

Then she added, "It would explain to me why my mother died, and it would allow me to be here for my children."

This single answer changed the way I think. I didn't grow up in a family with cancer. I was getting an inside clue of what this is all about.

As we stood in the parking lot at Universal Studios, Tiffany asked, "Are you on Facebook?"

I asked her, "What's Facebook?" (That was before everyone

knew about Facebook.) I got home, and I created a Facebook account and started a Facebook group: LearnAboutHBOC.

Next, Tiffany called me and said, "Is there anybody who could help us get this story out to the public?"

Advocacy!

One of her high-school friends, Christine, messaged back, "I work for Comcast Cable in Philadelphia[48], and if you make commercials, we'll put them on."

So we made commercials. They were really bad. What do doctors and patients know about making commercials anyway? A company called MacGuffin Films stepped up and took on the project. MacGuffin makes national commercials: Olive Garden, McDonalds, CableVision. They took us to Silver Cup Studios where they filmed "30 Rock" and "The Sopranos" in New York. "30 Rock" filmed the day we were there.[49]

We made three commercials. We couldn't understand why they would spend $80,000 to $100,000 to make them for us, because that's what it costs to make real commercials. Near the end of the day, they told us they just had a makeup artist who was twenty-eight or twenty-nine years old who died from breast cancer. They had never heard of BRCA testing.

Christine from Comcast put our commercials on the air. I didn't get to see them because they were on in Philadelphia, but she pushed the agenda. "I spoke to Comcast in New England, and I spoke to Comcast Northwest."

They ended up airing on NBC in Washington D.C., in Washington State and from Maine to Florida. Next, Christine e-mailed that we got a big one, WABC-TV in New York. ABC showed them during "Regis" and during "The View," and we got hundreds and hundreds of calls after that.

My kids thought I was cool because the PSAs started showing up between innings of the Yankees and Mets games. The Yankees showed them all the way through the World Series that year.

One day, I came to labor and delivery, and one of the female OB/GYNs teased me. "Last night, what you were doing in my bedroom? I was lying in bed, and all of a sudden, I heard you talking to me. I look up at the TV, and there you were."

I love that story.

Your BRCA patients, like Tiffany, will become advocates.

Voices from the Crowd

Lita Poehlman

Tiffany, when I got to the end of your story, I broke out in cold chills and just couldn't hold back the tears. My pathology report after my PBM showed I was one stage from breast cancer. Still, we were so lucky, because the timing of our situation was lifesaving.

Bless you, sweet girl, with a long healthy life filled with memories of all the wonderful *Simchas* (happy occasions) your mom couldn't be her to enjoy. She is watching and loving you all from a very special place.

Raechel Maki
An Offer to Help

It truly helps to have others who understand exactly what you're going through because they have been there. I saw my breast surgeon this week and offered to talk to other BRCA patients she had, if they need someone to talk to. She sounded very interested, so it makes me feel better that we are raising awareness and offering support across the country. Especially in smaller communities like mine, where large medical centers are not readily available.

Dr. Herman
A Side Point

It's a principle: If you work with five or more practitioners, there is someone in your office who qualifies for BRCA counseling and testing. Often we don't even know our employees' medical histories.

DR.SHEILA K.'S STORY

The Whole Story

Dr. Sheila K.
BRCA Testing Saved My Life

I will backtrack a little bit. Years ago, when BRCA testing first came out, we toyed with the idea of my having the test.

Every woman in my father's family (his mother and all her sisters) had breast cancer. While I didn't have all the details, I knew my paternal grandmother had breast cancer, but she didn't die from it. My paternal grandfather also had it but it was attributed to the estrogen he took for his benign prostatic hypertrophy. It also was not his cause of death. At that time, (I was in my thirties), the thought was that I was not going to do more with the knowledge, since I already did self-examination, yearly mammograms and sonograms.

I don't even think that breast MRIs were being done yet. One of my mother's sisters had breast cancer (after age fifty) and then a female cousin on my mother's side (not a daughter of the aforementioned aunt) also got treated for breast cancer. She was the first in my family I knew who got tested, and she tested negative.

Sheila's Red Flags

Family Members with Breast Cancer

Paternal Grandmother
Paternal Grandfather
Paternal Aunts
Maternal aunt
Maternal 1st cousin, BRCA negative

In February 2011, I got a call from one of my father's first cousins (DB). My father had passed a number of years prior. He and his sister (AB) were recently tested, because their mother (my paternal grandmother's sister) had died in her forties, of ovarian cancer. I hadn't known about that. Since they were positive for the BRCA1 mutation, they alerted the rest of the family and recommended we all get tested. Cousin DB's daughter was also positive, as was one of cousin AB's daughters. DB provided me with his test results and the family pedigree, a geneticist's dream for an inheritable disease, with the presumption my grandmother and all her sisters carried the mutation.

Armed with this information, I had no trouble having my health insurance cover the test, which I would have paid for anyway. My husband is a gyn, so we took the blood through his office.

Father's male 1st cousin DB	*BRCA1 positive*
Father's female 1st cousin AB	*BRCA1 positive*
Paternal grandmother's sister (great aunt)	*ovarian cancer*
DB's daughter	*BRCA1 positive*
AB's daughter	*BRCA1 positive*

I really wasn't too concerned about the results, figuring I would be positive but would deal with it when they came in.

The day they came in, my husband called from his office to give me the results. I wasn't too upset and found I had to console him more than myself. I had already thought about what I would do and, to me, it was an easy decision.

By then, I was forty-eight years old and had been experiencing hot flashes and some peri-menopausal symptoms. So getting rid of the ovaries was a no brainer. I had just started in a new practice in February and had plans to travel to Israel for two weeks in May. So I planned to do prophylactic oophorectomy in October. I would do it laparoscopically, be home that day, and back to work in a week. I had plans to do the mastectomy, but I couldn't take that much time off, so I would just increase my surveillance--add an MRI six months after my mammo/sono--and eventually have them done, as well. I was healthy and feeling great, in the best physical shape I had been in years. I arranged to start the workup--a pelvic ultrasound--for my prophylactic oophorectomy the week after I returned from Israel. I also scheduled an appointment with the GYN/ONC who we wanted to perform the surgery. This was the first week of June 2011.

On ultrasound, they saw what looked to be a large cyst (ten centimeters) on or around one of my ovaries. I was not concerned, since I had tied my tubes in the past, and we thought it could be fluid that built up in the tube. The week afterward, I saw the GYN/ONC. She discussed doing the surgery via the laparoscope, but didn't want to wait until October; she wanted to schedule it sooner.

We discussed all the implications of prophylactic oophorectomy and even with the cyst, she felt that we would be able to have it done in a minimally invasive way. Then, she examined me. She felt fullness behind my uterus and made the decision to get an MRI to further define the cyst and see what else might be going on inside my pelvis. One week later, I had my pelvic MRI. And then I received the call from the oncologist.

The findings on MRI were "concerning" (code for cancer) and she was scheduling my surgery to be done in two weeks. Also, she needed to do a laparotomy and lymph node biopsies, so I needed to plan to be in the hospital for three to four days and out of work for at least one month. Also, chemotherapy was most likely in my future, but we would meet the medical oncologist once we had the pathology reports from my surgery.

Wow! I had cancer! Ovarian cancer, no less, and not a single symptom! It was hard to believe, but it was true. I was one of the twenty-seven to forty-four percent of women with BRCA1 mutations who develop ovarian cancer, and I was not yet forty-nine years old.

I had my surgery, a TAH-BSO and lymph node biopsies on July 6, 2011. My surgeon was pleased with the surgery, but she apologized for the cut, which went from my sternum to my pelvis! She dissected lymph nodes all the way to my diaphragm, next to my kidneys and all throughout my abdomen. I had cancer on the outside of my bladder wall and outside my bowels that were adjacent to my ovaries. I had cancer in the fluid that built up in my pelvis. Thankfully, all my lymph nodes were negative and there was no obvious cancer past my pelvis.

I recovered well from my surgery, and I even went home after only two days. I met with the medical oncologist. We put a Mediport[50] and I started my chemotherapy on August 9, 2011. I received weekly chemo for eighteen weeks and am happy to report I tolerated it well. While still receiving chemotherapy, I went back to work the first week of October, because it was absolutely necessary for my mental health.

One year later, all signs of cancer are gone. I have been maintained on Avastin, which I receive every three weeks and have only three treatments left. My hair has returned as has my taste and my overall energy.

I know that having done the BRCA test and finding out I was positive was a lifesaver for me. With ovarian cancer, often there are no or very vague symptoms until the disease gets more advanced, and then the prognosis is worse. I may not have found the cancer had I not been planning on the surgery and the available screening for ovarian cancer is not very good.

My sister also tested BRCA1 positive, and she was able to have her surgery done as a preventive measure. I will eventually do the mastectomy. Hopefully, it will be done as a preventative procedure, when my oncologist gives me the okay. In the meantime, I am feeling great, continuing with my self-examinations, and doing my mammogram/ultrasound alternating with breast MRI every six months.

I am hoping my story will encourage you to go out and test your patients if they have these cancers in their family.

Knowledge was a lifesaver for me!

I am forever grateful to my father's cousins for alerting us to this family trait and giving me the information I needed to make a lifesaving decision for myself in regard to my health.

P.S. *It's now eighteen months later, CA-125–negative, CT-negative.*

Voices from the Crowd

Gail Mankiewicz

Thanks for sharing your letter, Sheila, and thank God for your cousins' concern for their relatives; my relatives seemed to just brush it off.

Dave B. (BRCA1-Positive Male)

Sheila is my wonderful, amazing cousin. When I told her about the BRCA1 gene mutation that runs in our family, she got tested. When she found out she was BRCA1 positive, her doctors discovered ovarian cancer in its earlier stages, so she was able to beat it. Way to go, Sheila.

This is why it is so important to spread the word. Knowledge is power. Sheila is living proof that you can make a difference in someone's life.

Janine
I Was Urged to Test

Thanks, breast surgeon. I was told about BRCA by my breast surgeon and urged to test. She did explain my options of bilateral PM. I think I was her fifth or sixth BRCA patient. She also told me about my ovarian cancer risk. When I asked her what surveillance my siblings should be doing if they don't get tested, she replied, "They should all get tested."

She has strong feelings about that! She has posters on the walls warning about hereditary cancer.

Randi Shapiro
How Your Office Could be Better

Dear Dr. J. S. breast surgeon, I want to thank you for being the first step in my BRCA journey these past three years. I appreciated your nonchalant attitude and making me feel that everything is one step at a time. When you tested me for the mutation, you felt there wasn't a strong enough history for me to even have it. To both of our surprise, it came back positive and your to-the-point advice was helpful and needed. I liked that you were never beating around the bush and told me exactly what I needed to hear.

Although I was very happy with how you and I have grown in our patient/doctor relationship, I was very unhappy with the way my results were given to me. At first, I was never called with an answer and had to hound your office for the results. After I finally got someone to tell me what it said, all they would say to me was it came up with "deleterious mutation." After asking what that meant, the woman said she didn't know and just told me to call so-and-so (genetic counselor). Being unfamiliar with the wording and the importance of knowing what it meant I felt it was no big deal. I didn't rush to speak with a genetic counselor, and I even considered thinking that it was negative. I didn't think an appointment with someone to tell me negative results was worth my time.

When I decided to go through with the appointment, months

later, just out of curiosity, I was floored that what I was told on the phone was actually a positive, and I should consider my options! I walked out of her office totally unprepared for what I had heard and could barely make it through the next few days. If I had been told by a doctor I had trusted and had a conversation with him (namely, you), I would have been more prepared and ultimately stronger with the blow I was hit with.

Aside from the experience of getting my results, I have been beyond happy in your care. I was confident in your reputation and in you that you would get every last piece of breast tissue there was. I am very happy with my end results, a year later, and in part, I am happy I had you to guide me through my journey.

Heather Millar
Why I Love My Surgeon

I have met a lot of doctors in the last two months, and I have met three beautiful, accomplished surgeons at three world-class cancer centers: NYU, Sloan Kettering[51], and UCSF[52]. I liked them all, but I love my surgeon at UCSF, Shelley (Eun-Sil) Hwang. Here's why Dr. Hwang rocks: Not even 48 hours after a friend of a friend sent her an email asking her to take me on as a patient, explaining I was in New York, moving to San Francisco in two weeks, Dr. Hwang calls me. She listens to my whole story, rather short at that time. She explains things. She tells me a little bit about herself.

Turns out her daughter went to preschool at my daughter's new school. We talk about a friend of mine who's written a book she admires. She asks if I am Chinese, since I spent time in China, and majored in Asian languages and history. I say no, European mongrel with Germanic, Anglo-Saxon overtones. She says that's kind of what she figured, given my last name is not very Chinese. We laugh.

She makes me feel hopeful and strong. Officially, I am not even her patient at this point. She is a surgeon! She is supposed to be brusque and brilliant, maybe not super good at people skills but great with a scalpel. She is supposed to be too busy for this kind of thing!

Dr. Hwang emails within the next week, saying she's been in touch with my doctor at NYU and with the doctor at Sloan Kettering, who gave me a second opinion (coincidentally, the doctor who trained her).

Just before we move, she sends me another email, saying she hopes I'm coping okay during such a period of change.

She calls two days after we get to California, says she wants to move up my consultation so we can do surgery as soon as possible. "We're going to take care of this," she says. "I'm so glad you waited to have the surgery here, but the waiting must have been hard. You can take a break from being strong for a while."

When we meet her, three days after arriving in San Francisco, the first thing she does is give me a hug. She is warm, and smart, and thorough. I feel like I've known her a lot longer than two minutes.

On the day of surgery, I do not see her while I am conscious. I almost fainted and threw off the schedule, and I bet she has a few fires to put out as a result. She comes into the OR after I've gone off to happy land.

I get out of the recovery ward pretty quickly. With the motivation of my sister-in-law's enchiladas, I make it a point to walk and pee as quickly as I can. We're just pulling into the garage at our temporary apartment building when my iPhone rings. "Hi, it's Dr. Hwang. I wanted to see you before you left but you got out of there fast!"

She tells me the surgery went well. They took out a piece about five centimeters by two centimeters. "I was afraid that if we had to go in again, you'd want to just take the whole thing off. I don't think that's necessary at this point."

How does she know me so well, so quickly? I tease her about her incredibly handsome surgery fellow. She says I sound really good for someone who's just had surgery. Again, she makes me feel strong and hopeful.

Dr. Hwang has a reputation for really caring about her patients, for going to bat for them, for being so, so good at what she does.

She seems detail-oriented, but not so rigid that she liked living in control-crazy Singapore (where there's a fine for not pulling the toilet chain, and for throwing gum on the street). After she finished her training, she went to Singapore for a year, but came back to California. A woman after my own heart.

~~Heather had breast cancer. She was diagnosed at forty-seven, and is now forty-nine. She has finished active treatment, two surgeries, chemo, radiation, monoclonal antibodies. These days, she only takes medication to suppress her uptake of estrogen, since her tumor was highly reactive to that hormone.

Voices from the Crowd

Kay Edwards

I was seen by a breast nurse the day after my mastectomy, when I was high as a kite on morphine. Because I could move both arms, she never came back. I had no advice about the help and support available.

Teri

I guess we've all had our share of bad experiences! On the plus side, I've also been treated with care and kindness too.

Where I had my PBM, in New Orleans, the hospital was staffed with a lot of breast cancer survivors, and one day my nurse was a Previvor, too! I mentioned to my doctor how impressed I was with how compassionate everyone was (right down to the janitorial staff!) and he said that he treats his patients how he'd want his wife to be treated, if she were going through this. Wish all doctors would look at it like this.

Letters to Gynecologists & General Practitioners

Helen Smith
Thanks Ob/Gyn

Interestingly enough, my OB/GYN actually brought up the BRCA test to me. Fast forward a year later, glad I did it, and I'm really glad that I know!

Tina
Thanks for Listening

Dear current GP, the biggest thing you have done is support me in my request for BRCA testing. This has not only saved me from breast cancer recurrence, but because of this knowledge, I have been able to reduce my chances of ovarian cancer. In agreeing to support me in this testing, you have also had a massive impact on my daughter's life and health, as she has been able to also be tested. Being BRCA2 positive is empowering for both me and my daughter. I will be forever grateful.

I have to say, you actively listen, respond, and if you are unsure, you are honest. You get back to me when you have done research and speak/share the information in a way that encourages and affirms decisions I make. I could not ask for anything more in a GP. Thank you.

Krystal Mikita

Dear Plastic Surgeon, from the moment I heard you speak, I knew you were the doctor for me. Deciding to remove the only parts of my body I was ever comfortable with and confident about was not an easy decision to make. During our first consultation, you gave me the reassurance I needed, that any woman would need, especially being a single woman in her twenties. I was terrified, but you answered all of my questions in a way that helped to reaffirm my decision to follow through with this risk-reducing surgery. After my surgery, I was expecting to have my follow up appointments with either you or the close colleagues I had met and established a good rapport with. Through the first stage, I felt very well taken care of and that I was in great hands. I only wish my good feelings had remained throughout my entire experience, and not just at the beginning.

When I had revision surgery, things went wrong. I had complications, but I never saw you. Every time I had an appointment scheduled with you, I only saw your colleagues or strangers (to me) who were your fellows and only with you for a short time.

I choose *you* as my doctor for a reason. When I expressed my concerns to them, they would brush me off, essentially telling me I'm silly. I know you're a busy doctor, and you have a lot of patients, but it would be great to see you more than just immediately after my surgery. The last fellow of yours I saw highly lacked any bedside manner or tact, and I left that appointment feeling belittled and doubting everything I'd done. Don't get me wrong, I love the reconstruction you did, and think you are a wonderful surgeon, but I feel you dropped the ball as far as being personally involved in my follow-up care.

Mary S.
Forty-Seven-Year-Old Breast Cancer Survivor
BRCA-Positive

Dear Former Gynecologist, I have to tell you, I am angry with you. I came to your office three years ago for a checkup. At that visit, I told you my father's mother, my grandmother, had breast cancer and that my father's sister died from ovarian cancer. You told me not to worry, as these cancers were not on my mother's side.

Well, that was a big mistake. I have now been diagnosed with breast cancer myself, and I never should have gotten it.

My new doctor tested me and determined I am BRCA positive and it came from my father's side of the family. I would have taken measures, had I known three years back. It was a no brainer for me. I would have had my breasts off in a second and avoided the cancer I have today. Now, I have to have chemo and who knows what is next. I don't want to think about it.

So my advice to you: don't blow off the next woman who comes in with a similar history. BRCA comes through the father's side like it does through the mother.

Just thought I would let you know.

Katrina W.
Practice Good Medicine

Dear NP, when I was crying in your office asking you about breast cancer screening and genetic testing and when you referred to it as the "cut and burn route," I was floored. But because I was persistent, you agreed I should, "talk to someone in genetics." However, when you came back with, "My friend said you're not high risk," and, "Start shopping at the Whole Foods," I realized you are an idiot who was letting your personal opinion affect my health. Matters like this should not be left up to your personal opinion.

Mary B.

My main message for providers is: Please listen to patients' questions and concerns and then answer, respond, research and provide follow-up as appropriate. Please always review patient histories verbally with your patients.

Despite working as an RN, I still fall into the patient trap. We, as patients, tend to think if we've filled out all the forms and/ or asked questions, if the physician failed to address something, it must not be important. If the physician isn't worried, why should we be? If our concerns get shot down or our needs aren't getting met, why should we keep taking time off of work, sit in the waiting room for an hour or more, and then pay a physician to do nothing for us? Honestly, that's what it feels like too often.

Prior to my BRCA testing, I went to my breast care center armed with the knowledge that five physicians and one genetic counselor had all told my twin sister (after her first breast cancer was found) that she was BRCA2 positive, and I had a copy of her lab work with me. The NP read the lab report (which showed positive for deleterious mutation) and said, "Well, at least she doesn't have BRCA, and you don't need to be tested."

My immediate thought was, "I must be stupid." I didn't question the NP. When my sisters heard what the NP said, they immediately corrected me, and my PCP ordered the screening test. I feel that providers expect compliance from their patients, but in turn, we would really appreciate competence. And courtesy, compassion, communication, professionalism...

DeAnna Howe Rice
The Urgency of Testing

Dear Physician, for hereditary breast and ovarian cancer patients carrying the BRCA genetic mutation, our risk as women goes up to eighty-plus percent that we will develop cancer in our lifetime. It is a staggering statistic. For the majority of carriers, this means that, unless we die from an accident or other means before we are diagnosed with cancer, it will be the only way to avoid the diagnosis. To have any chance of survival, we must be tested and educated about early detection and risk reducing measures.

Voices from the Crowd

L.
Dear Plastic Surgeon

"Dr. Jack," my surgical results were less than perfect, but I was so relieved to have reduced my risk that I did not worry too much about that until years later. As I obtained routine health care over the years, I found the knowledge of various MDs regarding BRCA is highly variable.

I am a doctor myself, and I am still working on how to tactfully teach those who are less informed without bruising egos. I am also thrilled my current OB/GYN seems to know his stuff, and he also knows he can tell any of his patients to call me if they need peer support.

Raechel Maki

I must thank my primary care physician for being on top of things and listening to the severe concern and fear my sister and I had about developing ovarian cancer. Without her, we'd just being going along through life until that devastating day we get sat down in the little room and told, "You have cancer."

DeAnna Howe Rice
Early Identification

The number of people with a genetic mutation is relatively low for the general population (I've heard it's 1/500 people for BRCA). But for those of us carrying a mutation, just knowing you are a carrier is the key to life. When identified early, the knowledge gives us the power to avoid developing that first, second, third, or more cancers in our lifetime.

Debbie C.
My Team

Dear genetic counseling team, I was blessed because I was able to go to the UCLA High Risk Program[53] for women who are BRCA Positive. They have a whole team who walked me through the process and it began with a genetic counseling session and then the blood test. I felt supported through the genetic counseling process and was even able to email the genetic counselor with questions. All the consequences were discussed with me, and I left with pages and pages of information. My insurance covered the testing fees and also covered my bilateral mastectomy and reconstruction. I am still waiting to see if they will pay for the tattooing.

Alice D.
RE: Debbie's Letter

It would be great if these teams were available to everyone. It seems that, in most places in the US, like here in Fergus Falls, Minnesota, you can't get that same care you got in UCLA. Yes, you were blessed.

Amanda Herrick
England, Great Follow Through

Dear Doctor Q and Mr. G. (Consultant Clinical Geneticist),

Thank you for taking an enormous interest in my family history and for considering my emotional wellbeing from the first day we met. You were adamant that, due to my family history, I should be tested for the BRCA mutation at my earliest convenience. Upon your kind insistence, I proceeded with genetic testing, resulting in a positive test result.

I thank you for your patience and understanding and for the many hours you offered afterwards to discuss the options available to me. You were kind enough to explain in great detail what having a positive BRCA mutation meant and how it would impact my life as I knew it by answering questions and allowing me to voice my feelings of anger, frustration and panic on almost every visit!

You introduced me to a genetic counselor, who, on more than one occasion, came to my home to discuss my options again but just as importantly to check on my emotional wellbeing, which I can honestly admit was a little unstable due to the emotional overload I felt had been dumped on me. I was thirty-four years old with three young children and had recently lost my mum to cancer, so at this time, I was certainly in no position to consider surgery whilst dealing with the aftermath of my new BRCA mutation knowledge.

You continuously kept the lines of communication open to me. You referred me to my local breast clinic and offered me both breast and ovarian screening with the option of discussing a mastectomy at a time when I was ready, thus eliminating scare tactics and pressure to go ahead with surgery before I was ready to do so.

Shortly afterward, I made a decision to relocate, and my only regret was knowing you were no longer going to be my consultant. My greatest concern was not having the support mechanism you had both given me since my initial diagnosis. However, once again you surpassed yourself by referring me to another amazing team of geneticists in what was then the beginning of a new chapter in my life. Within weeks of relocating, I had already received communication from not only a new consultant clinical geneticist, but also a warm and welcoming letter from a new Macmillan genetic nurse, who arranged appointments for me to continue discussions about preventative surgery.

At no time did I ever feel alone; neither did I ever feel I would make these life-changing decisions without the support of my medical team. Obviously, since we last spoke, you probably won't be surprised to learn my surgeries are complete, but without your constant support and patience, I certainly don't feel I would be where I am. I can only reiterate how blessed I feel to have been given the foundations needed to make my own life changing decisions. Your gift of knowledge has not only helped me adjust to a life with BRCA but you have also helped me in my journey to improve the lives of other BRCA patients who might need the same support I was offered.

Voices from the Crowd

Pat Martin

I am fifty-one and was feeling so fortunate to not have developed cancer yet. When I went for my annual mammogram this summer, I asked them about testing. They referred me to a genetic counselor, who walked me right in! I am so thankful for her caring and giving attitude. My brother felt I would be negative, since I am already fifty-one. He felt he would be positive. But as it turned out he is negative (thank God), and I am the positive one.

Jane Waldbaum

I put my own team together. The genetic counselor helped me so much with the testing part, but she didn't really know anything too much about the different breast reconstruction procedures and the surgery for the ovaries. So I found a great surgeon and plastic surgeon, plus my gyn went over the BSO and menopause issues with me.

Dorit Amikam

As a scientist, a molecular oncologist and a genetic counselor, I always invited my families in which a mutation for a hereditary cancer (colon/breast and other) was detected, for several sessions, as many as they need. Hereditary cancer was an integral and dominant part of my lectures in my courses in the medical school, and international conferences. It is surprising how knowledge is limited. Therefore, our work is cut out for all of us.

Teri

My genetic counselors shared some information with me about why they felt I should have my breasts removed, too. Though initially based on my personal family history, I was only going to have the hyst/ooph. The idea that cancer could grow so drastically in a BRCA mutant in between check-ups, even those done regularly, every six months, scared the daylights out of me. The fear of that outweighed my fear of having the double mastectomy.

Letters to Plastic Surgeons

Nicki Boscia Durlester
With Gratitude and Respect

Dear Dr. Orringer, just when I thought I could not possibly go to another doctor's office and fill out forms, I found myself in the happiest place on earth, also known as Dr. Jay Orringer's Beverly Hills Plastic Surgery Center.[54] At 2:00p.m. on April 2, 2009, I met an incredible doctor and extraordinary man. You changed the direction of my psyche after my stage IIA breast cancer diagnosis and added some much needed levity to an overwhelming situation. You would also put me back together and make me physically whole again.

When you walked out to the waiting room to greet me, you shook my hand with both of yours and led me to your office with tender loving care. We sat and talked for hours while you explained exactly what would happen during my bilateral mastectomy. My breast surgeon would remove my breasts and you would immediately begin reconstruction. I would not leave the hospital disfigured as my mother had decades before after her radical mastectomy. You showed me your work and it was clear to me you were a gifted surgeon and a true artist who cared deeply about your patients. I was so convinced you were the right plastic surgeon for me that I did not seek a second opinion. That spoke volumes, since typically, I have a need for several opinions and get mired in analysis paralysis.

I could not have made a better decision. In the days after I was discharged from the hospital, following my bilateral mastectomy and reconstruction with expanders, you made house calls to check on me and remove my drains. You gave me your cell phone number so I could reach you anytime, day or night. You were always accessible throughout the fill process, exchange surgery, nipple and areola reconstruction. Moreover, I had zero complications throughout the entire process. I did not realize how important the plastic surgeon would be when I was first diagnosed. I spent more time with you than my breast surgeon or my oncologist. I cannot imagine haven taken that journey with anyone else.

Thank you, Dr. Orringer, for your old-world sensibilities and your state-of-the-art surgical skills. You are a *mensch*[1] of a man, and I am hugely blessed you are my plastic surgeon. One in a million!

Marianne Hudson
RE: Nicki's Letter

Chills! We all hope and wish for that kind of compassion within our doctors. Dr. Orringer: Can you come to the East Coast? Pretty please?

From An Anonymous Patient

Hi, Teri, I hope you are well. I'm no writer, and I've taken a few days to think about what I would like to say. I'm going to

---

[1] *From about.com/Judaism, mensch is a Yiddish word that means, "a person of integrity." A mensch is someone who is responsible, has a sense of right and wrong and is the sort of person other people look up to. In English, the word has come to mean "a good guy."*

try and write this without crying. (*Ha-ha!*)

Dear Doctor, I can't begin to thank you enough for what you have done for me. You were on my side from day one. We were on the same team and together we fought this bullshit! Your skills are incredible, and there is and was nobody else I would allow to operate on me.

Things started to go wrong though. When, after ten days, I was readmitted with infection, the hand you gently placed on top of my foot while I cried meant a lot. You reassured me that you would make everything okay, and I put things in your hands.

The problem is this: When I was coming to the clinic every week because healing was so slow, you broke my heart telling me to give it one more week. I had a hole in my heart and I didn't want to give it time! I wish you had looked into my eyes and seen my pain. I wish you had seen I was weakening and needed your help. I wish you could have seen me come home to sit on my doorstep afraid to go inside for fear the tears would come and never stop.

I was alone and dying inside. All I ask is this, carry on being a wonderful doctor but look into the eyes of a person and ask this question. "What can I do to make things better for you to-day?"

Teri

I find this to be so heartbreaking. I also went through complications with my surgeries, and had post-op depression. It's very common, but not talked about much. I think it would be a great idea if our surgeons could have a list of counselors on file to help us with our emotional issues as well as our physical issues. The process of a mastectomy or oophorectomy is an emotional as well as a physical change, and it would be nice if the emotional aspect were addressed as well.

Eve Wallinga
Non-BRCA-Positive Breast Cancer Survivor

To the local reconstructive surgeon, I want to thank you for agreeing to squeeze me in during those days of panic, to explain to me that it was possible I could wake up from the mastectomy with a replacement breast. I'm very disappointed that the only techniques you offered were implants or a TRAM flap. Though you did mention free flap reconstruction (which not all plastic surgeons will even tell their patients about), you told me so with a curled lip, discouraging me, and then telling me that after such a procedure, the whole thing could just die, leaving me nothing. I had a right to objective information, not to feel limited by what you could do for me.

Thank you, God, for scrambling those reconstruction plans just prior to my surgery, so I'd have time to do my own research and ultimately choose a different procedure that did require my traveling out of state, but ended up providing me a beautiful, living breast. It was hard to live with the flat chest for a few months, but the wait was worth it.

To my fabulous breast reconstruction surgeons, you did such an amazing job the first time around, I was able to just focus on my heightened risk for cancer recurrence, while making my difficult decision with minimal aesthetic concerns. Also, it made the prospect of going through it all over again something I could contemplate, knowing I'd come through it fine before, even though we did encounter a bit of a bump along the road.

Anonymous

Dear Dr. S., (Plastic Surgeon),

You are worth your weight in gold! You took dead, cancer-ridden tissue off my body and replaced it so delicately with live tissue, giving me a tummy tuck at the same time. It wasn't easy, because radiation had fried the blood vessels, but you persisted. Twelve hours later, you didn't go home. You stayed. You were there when I came to. You were there a few hours later. You were there in the afternoon the next day. Only then did you crash for twenty-four hours. You limit breast reconstruction to one a week. You put your everything into the individual you are with for two days. You are awesome.

When you asked if I would be a contact for your future patients, I did not know it would open up doors to friendships and bonds with them. I feel honored and privileged in speaking to other women who are about to go through the same procedure. You are part of the team of medical professionals I feel trust their patients' intuition, decisions and create a feeling of empowerment at a time that is fragile and personal. Your manner is empowering.

Voices from the Crowd

Stephanie Bangel

There is so much more to these surgeries than the surgery itself. I am so happy to read about caring doctors who take the time before and after for the wellbeing of their patients.

Carol
Urge Your Patients to Get Tested

Dear Dr. T, we have known each other for quite some time. Since that dreadful day in 1996, when I was 36 and I came to see you after getting a biopsy report of some sort of metastatic mystery cancer in my right axilla. You were patient, optimistic, kind, and helpful in getting the ball rolling to initiate more extensive pathology studies. The result was what you suspected: an affected lymph node from breast cancer.

Given the clinical picture, my age and ethnic background, you treated me for stage II breast cancer, encouraged me with an optimistic prognosis, and continued to treat me with patience, respect, kindness, and optimism.

A few years later, you suggested I undergo BRCA testing, which was in its infancy. I told you I was reluctant. My ovaries had survived the onslaught of adjuvant chemotherapy and were still pumping estrogen that was hopefully keeping my heart healthy and definitely keeping my sex life healthy. I said I wasn't sure if I was ready to undergo the recommendations if it were positive. And you left it at that.

We had known each other a long time. You know I was a bit of a know-it-all. As a doctor, you knew how much I didn't know about this emerging field. If you had said, "Carol, you had a hard to detect malignancy, (now we know it was triple negative, a term we didn't even use in 1996), this malignancy occurred ten years earlier than when it struck and killed your paternal grandmother. I really urge you to have the test."

I would have done it. And, if I had, maybe I could have avoided a new case of breast cancer from rearing its ugly head at forty-nine. At the visit before my annual mammogram that year, I told you I was ready to have BRCA testing. My ovaries had retired. I was now ready to deal with the ramifications if the test was positive. But it was too late. Breast cancer had already struck again.

I did the test, of course, right away. The positive results helped me decide to undergo a double mastectomy instead of a single one. I am completely at peace with this decision. I parted with my ovaries a few months after completing an aggressive course of adjuvant chemotherapy in time for my fiftieth birthday.

It's not your fault my cancer came again. It's not your fault I didn't do the BRCA test earlier. It was my decision. You have always respected my intelligence and my autonomy. I do wish you had been just a little more insistent and pointed out all the reasons why I should. I am pretty sure I would have listened. I act like a know-it-all, but I know I'm really not. So if you happen to meet another know-it-all like me, share what you know with what she may not. Let her reach the decision. Please guide her to that decision with knowledge we have today.

Teri

Carol, thank you for sharing. Your story reminds me of something I've heard Dr. Herman say a few times. He goes around the country giving lectures to other doctors about BRCA stuff. One of the other doctors said to him (paraphrased as I don't recall exactly), "It's easy enough for you; your patients want to be tested. Mine don't."

Dr. Herman's response is, "Patients don't want to test but they will do it, if their doctor tells them it's important."

I like the example of the Pap smear. Who wants to go in for a Pap smear? Really, what woman wants to go through that? It's embarrassing, it's uncomfortable, but we do it because our doctors tell us we should do it. Same thing with the BRCA test, if our doctors stress the importance of it to us, then we'll do it. If he shrugs it off like it's no big deal, then we'll think it's no big deal, too. I wonder if doctors realize the power their words have over a patient.

Dr. Herman

Go, Teri! I couldn't agree with you more. We need to guide our patients with the best up-to-date medical knowledge.

Rosie G.
Teri's Mother

Dear Oncologist,

I have very few complaints about your care personally. You have been very caring and professional; you have never given up on me. The same cannot be said of your office staff, from your appointment secretary to your chemo nurse. They all are very badly in need of sensitivity training on how to best deal with cancer patients, especially those who have been fighting for many, many years.

Your cancer center should have started treating the entire patient, not just the tumor, years ago. We are not a tumor. We are people with tumors; the tumors affect the whole body, as does the treatment, so the whole body should be treated. We have mental, emotional, and physical side effects that also need to be treated. They are as serious as the tumors you are more concerned about.

All of this should come under the patients' insurance, as all the problems are caused by either the tumor or the treatment of them. The patient should have no out-of-pocket expenses other than the co-pay, if any.

Why should I, as the patient, have to call the chemo nurse for PET scan, blood work, etc., results every time, when she gets paid to call me?

When a patient calls to find out why her appointment has been re-scheduled for a month after the original date, when just finding out her cancer has recurred yet again, she was then accused of crying and screaming she needs to see the doctor. Insensitivity again! A little sensitivity goes a long way when working with people with terminal diseases!

I believe sensitivity training should be required for all medical staff, including doctors. We should be treated with respect and dignity!

My fight began on September 11, 2001 (The 9/11[55]), the day of my first surgery for advanced BRCA1-positive ovarian cancer. What a date to celebrate your life being saved while so many were lost! But out of the ashes, life shall begin.

We may not be in a foreign country fighting with guns, tanks, etc., but we are in a war, fighting for our lives every day. We suffer from PTSD just like a soldier fighting overseas for the same reasons, fighting with no end in sight. We fight twenty-four/seven/three-hundred-sixty-five days per year.

Teri

Mom, reading this choked me up and kind of pissed me off, too. I want to speak to that staff, but you won't let me. It's just not okay for them to treat their patients in this way. I wish you had more options where you live.

Thank you for taking the time to write this. I know you're having a rough time right now with the chemo, so I'm especially grateful to you for doing it. I love you!

Rosie G.

Thank you, Teri. It was hard for me to do this, but I know how important it is for us to get it out there. I love you, too!

Voices from the Crowd

Eve Wallinga

Thank you to the oncologist who finally actually took the time to read my records, test results, pathology report, reams of studies. Instead of treating me like a neurotic, ill-informed woman who had a sick desire for a prophylactic mastectomy, you treated me like an intelligent and thoughtful human being. You gave me the respect and support I was searching for during that time of terrible darkness, fear, and indecision. You are the best! A thousand times, thank you!

To all you oncologists: Please get some decent magazines in your waiting rooms. We are sitting out there trying to think about anything other than our own demise. Sports magazines or two-year-old cast-offs from your home subscriptions just don't cut it!

Raechel Maki

None of what they were offering sounded like a guarantee. I would be okay except the surgical side, which, at the time sounded really radical to me. That's when I dove into researching BRCA and consulted with oncologists. What changed my mind about the surgeries was having my oncologist tell me that, if I were his wife, his daughter, his sister, surgical removal of the tissues was the best, and in his mind, the only good option to save my life.

Letters from Doctors

Bob Rankin
M.D., Pittsburgh, Pa. — October 28, 2010

Not many physicians know about testing. My positive test was on a patient who had breast cancer seventeen years ago. I just operated on her for a pelvic mass, which turned out to be stage IA cancer of the ovary. I got the genetic test post-op and it was positive. I sent the results on to the oncologist since I thought he might be interested. He called to ask me what the results meant. Her son is an oncology fellow and he was unaware of the testing either.

~~Dr. Rankin completed his residency in obstetrics and gynecology at the University of Maryland. He is board certified in Obstetrics and Gynecology. Dr. Rankin has practiced in Mt. Lebanon since 1981.[56]

Dr. Herman

Dr. Rankin, thank you for your letter. I have had a similar experience. I met with a physician who found a BRCA mutation in one of his patients. He gave her the number for the oncologist. When the patient called to schedule an appointment, the receptionist wouldn't give her one. Why? Because the patient didn't have cancer and they only see cancer patients.

Donald W. Aptekar M.D. (Denver, CO)
Why I Test My Patients — April 23, 2009

My colleagues tell me it takes a lot of time and a lot of effort to do it! So why do I do what I do to identify and counsel patients at risk for hereditary breast and ovarian cancer?

Because it saves lives!

I have practiced OB/GYN for over thirty years. I have cared for a handful of patients, maybe six, who were diagnosed with and died from ovarian cancer. Three of them must have had BRCA mutations and could have been identified. I could have saved them and their families from a brutally awful death. I know this now from the current availability of testing which was not available in time for these women. I now care for their sisters, daughters, and sons, and I can be proactive in testing them and doing things to improve detection and prevention. Counseling and testing saves lives. It's proven.

Nothing in my specialty is worse than finding ovarian cancer in a patient. It is usually spread throughout the pelvis, and I know that, despite the best of care in treating this disease, we do not cure ovarian cancer in most cases. If I can identify those at greatest risk and offer them treatment that can save their lives, they are grateful beyond imagination.

Fear! I have spent many years caring for women who watched their mothers die at young ages of breast and ovarian cancer.

They live with the fear that they will contract this cancer but they don't know when. Tracing BRCA-positive families also allows me to identify those women who do not carry the gene mutation and therefore are at normal or slightly increased risk for developing these diseases. Finding negative test results in

daughters ages six, eight, and ten. Wow. Just think of what the implications of a missed positive test could have had on her life and family tree.

I ask myself what would have happened if I hadn't paid attention to that lecture. What if I had just kept going along like I had in the past?

This is not that complicated. I guess I am just a surgeon, simple minded at times. To me, it's clear: Every woman who meets criteria needs the test! How can I manage them without it? The implications are far-reaching, and that is where my counseling comes in.

Finally, it's my goal to educate surgeons on management of BRCA positive patients. This includes surveillance as well as proper, minimally-invasive surgical techniques. You just don't go in and "yank everything out."

"C" told me she just wanted to be around for her daughters and that the surgery had to be done. Thank you to BRCA for saving her life and for helping us monitor her three daughters.

James Kondrup, M.D. is an assistant clinical professor, Department of Ob/Gyn Upstate Medical Center; Syracuse, NY, Binghamton Campus[60] and is an international trainer on minimally invasive surgery for Ethicon Endo-Surgery[61].

Dr. Herman

What an interesting case and congratulations on picking up this BRCA-positive family. When you find one person, you find the whole family. Dr. K., you surely have changed the course of their healthcare and their lives.

Each year, in the United States, there are approximately sixty thousand cases of DCIS and the numbers have been rising. There are two reasons given for this increase.[62]

- *Women are living much longer. Age is the number-one risk factor for DCIS and breast cancer.*
- *More women are going for mammograms and the quality of the equipment has improved. Thus, with better screening, more DCIS is detected.*

What is the relationship of DCIS to BRCA? In 2005, in the *Journal of the American Medical Association,* Dr. Elizabeth B. Claus, MD, PhD et al wrote a paper called "Prevalence of BRCA1 and BRCA2 mutations in women diagnosed with ductal carcinoma in situ."[63] They reported on three-hundred-sixty-nine cases of DCIS and determined DCIS is part of HBOC. They concluded the findings suggest that, once an appropriate patient history or family history is present, the patient should be screened in a similar fashion to those with invasive breast cancer.

In other words, DCIS is a risk factor, a red flag, for HBOC.

Dr. Kondrup, you tested your patient appropriately. You are correct when you stated her sisters and eventually her daughters need to be tested. Now, I have a question for you: Have you determined which side of the family the mutation came from? Is it maternal or is it paternal in origin?

I suggest you bring one or both parents in for counseling and testing. Although you did not report on the patient's uncles, aunts, grandparents, cousins, don't let them fall through the cracks. Do a little detective work! Think about how many people may be saved because you advocated and tested.

Robert Michaelson, M.D. FACOG
Willow Grove, PA -March 8, 2010

My interest and support for BRCA testing is both professional and personal.

My cousin's wife developed a premenopausal ovarian malignancy at age forty-seven. During the fifteen years she lived with this disease (it became chronic), she was tested for the BRCA gene mutations. She was found to be positive. The testing was initiated because of her earlier-than-usual onset of ovarian cancer.

Although she never developed evidence of a breast malignancy, she encouraged her daughter to undergo testing.

My cousin's wife died before her second grandchild was born. Her daughter found out that she was positive for a BRCA1 mutation in the interval between pregnancies. Using this information, she accelerated her attempts to achieve a pregnancy. She conceived and successfully delivered a healthy daughter. When she completed lactation, she underwent conventional mammography and, she also underwent bilateral MRI imaging, which showed an early breast malignancy. Even retrospectively, the concurrent mammogram did not show the tumor.

Because of the breast findings, my cousin's daughter underwent chemotherapy, followed by bilateral mastectomy and reconstruction. Finally, she underwent laparoscopic BSO.

It is our belief that these therapies will be lifesaving and health restoring. We believe the breast malignancy would not have been found as early as it was, had she not been aware of her BRCA status. Thus, I continue to be an advocate for BRCA and other inheritable disease testing and hope that patients and their providers will recognize the importance of screening.

Dr. Michelson practices at Abington Primary Women's Health in Willow Grove, PA.[64]

Dr. Herman

As you may be aware, thinking about patients with ovarian cancer has changed over time. The National Comprehensive Cancer Network (NCCN) guidelines[65] suggest that any women with ovarian cancer, no matter what age at diagnosis, should be considered for genetic testing.

Voices from the Crowd

Gail Mankiewicz
RE: Dr. Rankin's Letters

This is unimaginable that an oncologist and a new soon-to-be doctor doing a fellowship wouldn't know about BRCA testing!

RE: Dr. Aptekar's Letter

Thank God for doctors such as this one. Shame on his colleagues who seemingly don't want to be bothered to take the time to do this lifesaving work. Guess they'd rather treat the cancer than the patients.

Rosie G.
RE: Dr. Rankin's Letter

That's just plain scary!

RE: Dr. Aptekar's Letter

We need doctors like him to lecture to his peers as well as students about the importance of BRCA testing! What a great tool he would be in spreading the word!

Teri in response to Rosie:

That's exactly what Dr. Herman does when he's not delivering babies. He flies all over the country giving lectures to other doctors about the importance of BRCA testing. The world needs more Dr. Hermans! That is what the entire purpose of this book is: To educate our doctors so they can take better care of their patients.

Lori Adelson
RE: Dr. Apetkar's Letter

Please tell Dr. Aptekar thank you. My own sister saved my life, so to speak, by giving me knowledge of our BRCA gene.

My niece's partner died less than two years ago, in her early sixties, of metastatic ovarian cancer that was overlooked, even though her son was BRCA1 positive, she'd had breast cancer in her thirties, and her mom had died young of "female cancer". Sometimes things right in our faces are missed. No more!

Dr. Sheila K.
Dr. Apetkar's Letter

As a pediatrician and BRCA1 mutation carrier, as well as an ovarian cancer survivor, I ask about cancer history when I take a family history. I often suggest a parent inform their own doctor or recommend a visit to a geneticist if the parents tell me that there is breast, ovarian and/or colon cancer (possible Lynch Syndrome) is in the family history. I have shared my story with my patients. I hope that I can make a difference for these families.

Lisa Marie Guzzardi
RE: Dr. Kondrup's Letter

Bravo James Kondrup! The BRCA world needs more M.D.s like you!

Gail Mankiewicz
RE: Dr. Kondrup's Letter

This really stands out to me. *"I ask myself what would have happened if I hadn't paid attention to that lecture? What if I had just kept going along like I had in the past? This is not complicated."*

It makes me wonder how many others in this field are asleep during the lectures and/or just don't give a damn.

I really appreciate this doctor's aggressive attitude toward testing patients for the BRCA genetic mutations. I'm sure that many lives are being spared. Thank you, Dr. Kondrup.

Lisa Marie Guzzardi
RE: Dr. Michelson's Letter

Kudos to Dr. Michelson! First for initiating BRCA testing on a forty-seven-year-old woman and then pursuing it with her daughter! The breast MRI continues to be the very best diagnostic tool for high-risk women. This woman was very, very fortunate to be in the care of a BRCA-savvy physician. How many women are not as fortunate?

Rosie G.
RE: Dr. Michelson's Letter

Boy, do we need more physicians like you!

FORCE
Facing Our Risk of Cancer Empowered

A Great Resource

Lisa Cohen
Founder and Executive Director–BRACHA.com

Israel: My mother, may her soul rest in peace, passed away in January 2006 at the age of age sixty-four of metastatic cancer that began as breast cancer. At the same time, my eldest sister, may her soul rest in peace, was ill with breast cancer. She subsequently passed away at the age of forty-four in March 2007.

Since my mother had become ill many years before, I knew in the back of my mind I had a somewhat higher risk of cancer, but apart from getting regular mammograms, it wasn't something I thought about. I believed that I had no control over getting cancer, so there was no point worrying about it. But then, after my mother passed away, my three healthy sisters did a genetic test. I didn't understand it from the little information that I gleaned by asking around. It sounded abhorrent and the prophylactic surgery that would be the result sounded like mutilation. I refused to do the test and reverted back to my beliefs that I have no control over whether I would get cancer.

Over the next six months, I felt a growing feeling of responsibility toward my three children and realized that, if there were something to do, I owed it to them to at least check it out.

I went for genetic counseling and came away much happier knowing that when they find I am not a carrier I would be able to stop all those horrible mammograms. But the result came back that I was positive. Since that moment, I have been through so many difficult situations and decisions and felt completely isolated throughout the whole process. Doctors gave short answers whilst looking at their computer screens. Cancer organizations didn't want to help. They would say, "You are not ill yet, dear."

My clinic had no idea who to refer me to. I had to push and fight every step of the way just to get information, and no one related to the emotions and complex decisions of the subject.

Only when I finally found the web site FORCE did I find the information I had been searching for. More importantly, I found a community. I was sponsored to attend the FORCE Conference last May, and there, I met so many wonderful people, all with, sadly, similar stories of losing family or themselves becoming ill at a young age. Everyone spoke freely about the decision-making process of BRCA carriers. It was truly an enlightening experience.

On my return to Israel, I realized how lucky I was to have been part of such an experience and wanted others in Israel also to have that opportunity to feel part of a community. I have been volunteering for the past six months in a high-risk clinic and have seen firsthand that an organization and website in Hebrew is needed. So I started one.

Thank you, FORCE.

Amy Shainman
FORCE Outreach Coordinator, Palm Beach County, FL

I want to tell you about FORCE, Lifesaving Support, Resources, and Information.

FORCE is the only national nonprofit organization devoted to individuals and families whose family history or genetic status puts them at high risk for ovarian and/or breast cancer.

I am a Previvor, someone who has never had cancer but has an extraordinarily high risk for getting the disease. The medical community uses the term "unaffected carrier" to describe individuals in this population, but that doesn't adequately capture the experience of those who face increased risk for cancer and their need to make difficult medical-management decisions. Although cancer Previvors face some of the same fears as cancer survivors, undergoing similar tests and confronting similar medical management issues, their emotional, medical, and privacy concerns are unique.

The term *Previvor* was coined in 2000 by FORCE[66], when women on the FORCE message boards struggled with how to identify themselves. These women weren't cancer survivors; they had never had the disease. However, they were part of an undefined group that needed a helpful label to ultimately identify themselves to their healthcare providers about their specific healthcare needs.

Ten years after FORCE created the term, Congress, under H.Res. 1522 (111th), recognized the unique challenges faced by women and men at high risk for cancer, declaring the last Wednesday of September every year as National Previvor Day, and establishing the last week of September as National Hereditary Breast and Ovarian Cancer Week to bridge the gap between Ovarian Cancer Awareness Month and Breast Cancer Awareness Month.[67]

What's my story? The family tree on my father's side is a road map for hereditary cancer. My grandmother, Lillian, died in 1934 at age thirty-three from breast cancer. Others on that side of the family had breast cancer, colon cancer, and ovarian cancer. However, we discovered this only when my sister, Jan, was diagnosed and treated for separate ovarian and uterine cancers in the fall of 2008. When she had genetic testing, we learned she carried a BRCA1 genetic mutation. We had heard of BRCA testing, but weren't aware of what it involved.

With all that my sister, Jan, learned from FORCE, after battling ovarian and uterine cancer, she decided to move forward with a prophylactic mastectomy and reconstruction. In preparation for her mastectomy, she had a breast MRI. The MRI and subsequent biopsy detected invasive ductal carcinoma. Her surgery was no longer prophylactic. Fortunately, her early stage had not spread. However, she endured several additional surgeries due to issues she encountered with reconstruction.

My own medical concerns started in 2009 when I tested positive for one of the three founder mutations associated with people of Ashkenazi Jewish descent. I inherited the genetic mutation from my dad, the same mutation my sister had inherited. What this meant was that, in my lifetime, I had up to an eighty-seven-percent chance of getting breast cancer and up to a fifty-percent risk of getting ovarian cancer (compared to the ten percent and four percent respectively of the normal population). However, in 2010, I chose to drastically reduce my cancer risk by having preventive surgeries. I had a prophylactic complete hysterectomy in March of 2010, and a bilateral skin-sparing, nipple-sparing mastectomy with implant reconstruction. I said good riddance to my ticking time bomb breast tissue and welcomed my new breasts and minimal scars. I became my own advocate, and ultimately, a pioneer in my family.

We didn't realize that different types of mutations had been identified in the BRCA1 and BRCA2 genes. We had no idea that being of Ashkenazi Jewish descent raises an eyebrow for concern. One of every forty Jewish people carries a BRCA1 or BRCA2 gene mutation. We didn't know that the different mutation types meant different things in terms of cancer risk.

We learned something hugely important: The idea that the breast cancer gene mutation can be only inherited from your mother, or her side of the family, is an epic misconception. A mutation can be passed to you from either your mother or your father; if either one have a mutation, you have a fifty percent chance of inheriting it.

I learned most about my BRCA1 genetic mutation from FORCE. Executive Director Sue Friedman founded the organization in 1999 on the principle that no one should face hereditary cancer alone. As a sixteen-year survivor of hereditary breast cancer, Sue knew that confronting cancer risk could be a complex, confusing, and highly individual journey. Sue has since co-authored the book, *Confronting Hereditary Breast and Ovarian Cancer: Identify Your Risk, Understand Your Options, Change Your Destiny.*[68]

Everyone's path is slightly different because there are no guaranteed prevention, screening, or treatment options. FORCE does not have definitive answers or medical solutions. Unfortunately, no one does at this time, but FORCE can help your patients navigate these uncharted waters by equipping them with resources, information, and support.

FORCE's mission is to improve the lives of individuals and families by providing support, education, awareness, advocacy, resources and research specific to hereditary cancer. Specifically, it was the 2010 annual Joining FORCEs conference in Orlando, Florida that provided Jan and me with invaluable information that helped us make important lifesaving decisions.[69]

Upcoming FORCE conferences will be held in Philadelphia. This change in venue is due to FORCE's exciting partnership with the newly created Basser Research Center at the University of Pennsylvania[70], which will focus solely on the prevention and treatment of cancers that are associated with inheritable BRCA mutations. This new center brings a new hope for future generations and the hereditary cancer community.

What I love about FORCE is the fundamental philosophy that knowledge is power.

FORCE wants everyone to be empowered to make the best healthcare decisions for themselves. On the FORCE website, you and your patients can learn all about hereditary cancer risk and get support, from talking with family members to cancer risk assessment, genetic counseling, risk management information, community privacy and discrimination laws, advocacy, research, and clinical trials. There are also message boards, chat rooms, and local community support groups.[71] More than that, FORCE has an extremely useful online patient experience tool and a gallery of members' post-mastectomy and reconstruction photos.

FORCE has empowered me to empower others. I am compelled to pay it forward by volunteering to be a FORCE outreach coordinator. I feel a responsibility to share my BRCA story and what I have learned about hereditary breast and ovarian cancer and BRCA gene mutations wherever and whenever I can, so that others can make the best healthcare decisions for themselves. My hope is that all women realize that knowing their family medical history and learning how they can stay healthy is the most loving thing they can do for themselves and their loved ones.

If you believe that breast or ovarian cancer runs in your family or your patient's family, strongly encourage them to contact a board-certified cancer genetic counselor, geneticist, or equally qualified healthcare provider. These experts can calculate a statistical range of risk for certain cancers. Counseling is extremely important in the genetic testing equation, especially for interpreting genetic testing results and identifying options. Even patients who test negative for a gene mutation need counseling about appropriate lifetime cancer screening and monitoring, as they may also have higher cancer risk than the general population.

To contact a qualified genetics expert, visit the FORCE website on genetic counseling or speak with a board-certified genetic counselor at FORCE's "Ask-A-Counselor" toll-free helpline (866-288-7475, ext. 704).

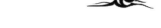

Voices from the Crowd

Marlene
When I Found Out

It was like a bolt of lightning struck me to the floor. I hung up the phone and cried so hard I could barely catch my breath. I had just turned forty. I couldn't get hold of my husband or my mother. I cried for at least an hour before I got the courage to look up support groups and found FORCE. I called the hotline and the founder, Sue Friedman, answered the phone. We talked for at least an hour. I felt so much better when I hung up the phone. I knew I had choices, but I knew there was no doubt I had to remove my breasts immediately. I knew that the ovaries would come out soon after the breasts. I was BRCA1 and over forty, I had to get the ball rolling.

Bee Urslv
FORCE Saved My Life

I found Sue from FORCE. She saved me. I still have her first email, and it makes me cry. I just reread it. The pain is right there. She emailed me on July 8, 2008 at 1:09 am and told me to breathe and that she would call. And she really did. Little ol' me, who was dying inside from frustration, isolation, and mixed messages. She told me where to find concrete research-based evidence and highly recommended a certified genetic counselor and counseling.

I started to focus and breathe again. She helped me find a clinic before she hung up the phone. What stranger takes time to care for someone else like that? A total stranger. She called me and we talked for an hour. I was astonished.

Teri to Bee

That is quite the story! I want to say, about Sue: She's wonderful, isn't she? I've also spoken to her on the phone many times over the years, and I know a few others who have, too. She really is that caring and genuine. I only hope to be even a fraction as helpful as she's been to the BRCA community. I do sort of have her up on a pedestal in my mind!

Amy Shainman
FORCE Outreach Coordinator, Palm Beach County, FL

When you need one-stop shopping, you go to Target. When you need one-stop information on hereditary cancer, you go to FORCE.

Amanda Herrick
BRCA and non-BRCA Cancer-Related Books

- *Pretty Is What Changes*, Jessica Queller
- *Eating Pomegranates*, Sarah Gabriel
- *I'm Still Standing*, Wendy Watson
- *Previvors*, Dina Roth Port
- *Why I Wore Lipstick to my Mastectomy*, Geralyn Lucas
- *Beyond the Pink Moon*, Nicki Boscia Durlester
- *Singing the Life*, Elizabeth Bryan
- *Positive Results*, Joi Morris and Dr. Ora Gordon
- *Pieces of Me, Genetically Flawed (Surviving the Breast Cancer I May Never Have)*, Veronica Neave
- *Promise Me*, Nancy G Brinker
- *Talk to the Headscarf*, Emma Hannigan
- *Now What?*, Amy Curran
- *The Premature Menopause Book*, Kathyrn Petras
- *Blood Matters: From Inherited Illness to Designer Babies, How the World and I Found Ourselves in the Future of the Gene*, Masha Gessen
- *How Connie Got Her Rack Back*, Constance Bramer
- *Staying Alive, A Family Memoir*, Janet Reibstein
- *Confronting Heredity Breast and Ovarian Cancer: Identify Your Risk, Understand Your Options, Change Your Destiny*, Sue Friedman.

- *The Pink Moon Lovelies: Empowering Stories of Survival*, Nicki Boscia Durlester
- *Make Mine a Double... A Mastectomy That Is*, by Beth Kaufman

Teri

When you need the support of a big sister, you can turn to the BRCA Sisterhood on Facebook.

SECTION THREE

Ideas
&
Thoughts

Our Friends, Relatives & Patients Speak

Bonnie Golden

The scariest word I can think of is cancer; however, cancer, to most of us, is just a word. When it happens to you or a loved one, the scariest word becomes the scariest time in your life, like it did for my mother, my family, and me.

Krystin Tate

We can't choose to be BRCA positive or not, but we can choose to become Previvors and live cancer-free and spread the word to save lives.

Jenny D.

I don't know if my story might touch or inspire you, but I do know that, with all of my heart, I have extended my own life by being pro-active and making hard choices to remove the parts of me that could potentially change my story away from something positive.

Teri

The burden of knowledge is a heavy weight to carry around. Other people can rally behind you, cheer you on and give you loving support. However, the only one who can truly carry this burden is the person with the mutation.

The decision to have prophylactic surgeries has been mine and mine alone. Yes, my husband and doctors have strongly encouraged me to have them, but all along, the choice has been mine. The hardest phone calls I've ever made are those that involved the scheduling of these surgeries. The calls were preluded by many months of anguish, fear, confusion, procrastination, research, learning, and mourning. I have gone through the stages of grieving[72]. I've been through denial, anger, bargaining, and depression. I've looped through them all more than once before I finally came to acceptance.

That has been the burden of knowledge for me, knowing that I have a genetic mutation that puts me in an extremely high cancer risk category, and knowing there is actually something I can do to take myself out of it. Unfortunately for me, it involves more than just eating a lot of broccoli, exercising regularly, and not smoking.

Margaret Tueller-Proffitt

Deep down in my DNA sits one mutated gene among thousands of normal, functioning genes. That gene has a name and a destiny to potentially spawn a deadly form of breast cancer and/or ovarian cancer. And this gene mutation doesn't discriminate.

Amy S.
Before BRCA Testing

We have all sorts of cancers in my family: colon, breast, ovarian, throat, lung, bone, stomach, and brain. I continually asked every physician I saw to order the BRCA testing, and was continually turned down. This past May, my OB/GYN finally agreed to order the testing, but told me it was unlikely I had the trait.

After BRCA Testing

The only thing I can think of at this moment is what I said to my OB/GYN, "Aren't you glad I pushed to get this test done? You sure would be feeling pretty bad if I ended up becoming a statistic, all because you didn't believe."

He agreed. I do think that, in the future, he'll be more likely to not dismiss a patient's desires/requests on this matter or others.

Kay Edwards

I look at things fairly positively. I am alive. I wouldn't be if I didn't have a family history.

Raechel Maki

I will not die as my mother did. She succumbed to ovarian cancer after a courageous and horrific four-year battle. Hers was a death I would not wish upon my worst enemy. I will most likely live to see my son get married and have children if he so chooses, yet another thing my mother was not privy to.

I will be here for my family, and God willing, will be here as a healthy individual, living a life that does not revolve around chemo treatments, CT scans, and days spent wondering when the cancer will come back.

Margaret Tueller-Proffitt

The gene mutation didn't care that my grandma couldn't attend my mom's wedding because she was too sick from cancer treatment. It didn't care that my mom's plate was already crowded with other serious physical, mental, and emotional challenges before she got her diagnosis. And it certainly didn't care that I'm happy, young, and want to use my ovaries and breasts to grow a large and healthy family.

Amy S.

The genetic nurse said because I wasn't sure exactly where my Jewish ancestors were from I didn't fall into the ratio that the hospital uses to tell if testing was warranted. Also because my sister, Kim, was the only one in the family under forty when diagnosed, she said Kim's cancers, breast and ovarian, were probably a fluke. It was hard to bite my tongue at that response.

Lulu Luke

In some ways, for many people with cancer who found out

they were gene mutation carriers, afterwards, it's like relief. It explains why you got breast cancer at the age of thirty-seven. On being BRCA positive: My family is very unusual in that we don't have a family history of much note of breast and ovarian cancer. I am the only one to have breast cancer, and there is one other who died at forty-five from ovarian cancer.

Dr. Herman

Lulu, you do have a strong history. One ovarian cancer makes it strong. One young breast cancer makes it strong.

Raechel Maki

To ignore the precious gift of knowledge we have been given would be like kicking my mother in the face and spitting on her fight.

Beth Weiner-Pfeiffer
Thankful for My Genes: A Thanksgiving Poem

I am thankful for my genes.
They made me what I am today.
I am cancer-free because I chose to know.
I am cancer-free because I chose to lose the parts that would give me trouble.
I am cancer-free because I chose life over death.
I am cancer-free because my genes don't control my life.
I chose to live.

Helen Smith

My mom really struggled to keep her life. She died of metastatic breast cancer. I told my husband and many friends when thinking of getting the testing done and my decisions to have the surgeries that someday I will die of something, but it won't be breast cancer!

Raechel Maki

I have a five-year-old son who I will be able to watch grow up, get married, and maybe have children, which are things my mother never had the chance to do. I am a Previvor and proud of it and would do it all again in a heartbeat to feel the relief I feel now, lying in my bed recovering from my surgery.

Tracy Layton

I already felt I knew my risk, but having the BRCA-positive result sends a red flag for your physicians to actually pay attention to nuances they might otherwise consider insignificant. I felt, before my mastectomy, that maybe, with the radiologist knowing my risk, he would be as vigilant as possible.

Raechel Maki

The genetic counselor actually said he was pretty confident I wouldn't have it. For some odd reason, I couldn't agree with him on that. In our family, if something bad can happen to you, it does. We occasionally joke that, "We are like the Kennedys, but without the money."

I just had this weird feeling when they drew my blood for the test that I would be positive. Can't really explain it, it was just there.

Sandra Lurie-Meir

I hate it when I have other women question why I am having prophylactic mastectomy done.

"You should not do it!"

"It is in G-d's hands."

"Your husband should divorce you."

They just don't get it! They can't grasp the concept that one must be proactive!

Amy S.

I basically have my sister to thank for bearing this burden of cancer to save my life. I'll get to be here to raise my two beautiful daughters without the looming cancer fairy over my shoulder all the time. She tells me all the time that if she had known we had this genetic flaw, she'd have done everything in her power to avoid cancer. She is my strongest backer of my upcoming surgeries. I feel guilty that I have this choice at my sister's misfortune, but she has told me that at least something positive is coming out of her cancer.

Teri

Sadly, Amy S.'s sister, Kim, lost her battle to cancer while we were writing this book.

Margaret Tueller-Proffitt

Dear Mom, remember when I was in sixth grade and kind of tubby and you brought me home a maternity dress and suggested I wear it to my first school dance? I forgive you.

Remember when you completely forgot my twenty-second birthday? I forgive you.

Remember when I had that baby cut out of my abdomen and you came and stayed in my four-hundred-square-foot apartment for four weeks to help? I forgive… I mean, thank you.

Remember when I was an embryo and you gave me that gene mutation that means I have a pretty good chance of getting breast cancer?

I forgive you.

And to be honest, it never occurred to me that you would require any sort of forgiveness. But when I think of my own children, the guilt I feel is enormous and surprising. And I find myself begging for their forgiveness because of this gene mutation, even though they are young. So I understand why you cried about this, and I want you to know that I forgive you, even though it might seem silly to do so and pray that my children can do the same, because that does not feel silly to me at all.

Love,
Your Genetically Mutated Daughter

Lulu Luke

People with cancer who tested positive have said to me, "I'd have been more surprised if I didn't have the gene." It's like they already know and the test is just confirmation.

Jean Haspel

I learned I had a high chance of recurrence of breast cancer. I immediately knew I was going to have to have a bilateral prophylactic mastectomy. I just did not know at the time how I was going to sell the idea to my husband. Luckily it was never an issue, and he has been loving and supportive throughout all the news and surgeries!

Raechel Maki

After my mother's death, I was a freakazoid about getting ovarian cancer. Every time I would go to my primary care physician for my yearly Pap/pelvic. My sister who sees the same doctor was the same way. She took a special interest in us after she had attended a conference about BRCA testing. I look at myself as lucky for once. If I didn't know about my BRCA status, I'd for sure get cancer at some point, because that's what happens to us in my family.

I try to think that everything happens for a reason. Maybe my mother's death, as horrible as it was, was not in vain. Now my sister and I have the opportunity to be there to see our children grow up and maybe have children of their own.

Amy S.

One week after testing, I received a call to make an immediate appointment with my OB/GYN. I am a BRCA1-mutation carrier. My sister, Kim, has yet to be tested. They are just assuming she has the same mutation, due to her having both premenopausal breast and ovarian cancers. My other sister refused testing and our brothers also have not been tested.

Sina Toscano

I am a BRCA parent as well as being BRCA1 positive myself. I have six daughters and the two who have tested are both positive, so that's one-hundred percent, so far.

Yes, it is a terrible burden, and the guilt sometimes hits, and all sorts of feelings emerge. In saying that, I don't blame my dad for passing the gene on to me, and really have never given it much thought. I have it and that is that. I know my girls feel the same, but yes, as a parent you can't help but wonder. As a parent with the gene fault, you know firsthand what is in store for your kids.

To know, at least, your daughter, like mine, is armed with a power that previous generations did not have means she has the choice to be proactive and at least prevent what might be, because, as you know, being BRCA positive it is not written in stone that you will get cancer, just your risk is higher.

Sharon Oisher-Stanley

I was being told that I had the BRCA1 mutation and the best thing I could do was do a prophylactic bilateral mastectomy, and I did not have cancer. I was literally blown away by this news. It was surreal. When I went to five more doctors who told me the same thing, it was even more shocking. My family could hardly believe it. My friends were stunned. Who does such a thing? Well, I did, and although I do not regret my decision, I regret that I had to remove one of the most beautiful parts of my body .

Teri

When I first tested for the mutation, I didn't know anything about it, other than what I read from my mom's positive BRCA1 test results. I had to figure a huge chunk of it out on my own. I had my husband--by alone, I mean, no other BRCA-positive people I could talk to. It was a scary place to be in and I swore I'd do whatever I could to make sure to help others, so that no one else would have to be as afraid as I was without having a safe place to share those fears. Hence, the beginning of the BRCA Sisterhood on Facebook.

Marlene

I found out my mom was positive first. I knew she would test positive, because she had breast cancer at twenty-seven and then again at thirty-eight. As soon as she gave me the news, I went to my doctor and had my blood drawn. I didn't want to wait for my genetic counselor appointment. Within two weeks, she called me and asked me to come in. I said, "Please, just tell me over the phone."

Rebecca Amy Stenning-White

I remember my fiancé coming 'round in the evening after I got my results and saying to me, "Everything is going to be okay."

I just shouted back at him, "Well, it's not going to be okay, is it? How can it be okay?"

He just stood there with tears in his eyes and didn't know what to say to me. It was an awful day, but I don't regret getting tested. I think no amount of counseling would have properly prepared me for a positive result.

Sharon Larsen

Having two aunts that had been diagnosed and since passed away from ovarian cancer and also my cousin having breast cancer, I bit the bullet two years ago and got tested.

To this day, I am thankful for my wonderful Aunty, who thought, "*Hmm*, maybe there is something genetically wrong in our family history." She got the ball rolling, got all the family history down and the testing on the way.

Cori Shade Williams

My aunt was tested in 2004, but I had to wait for my mother to be tested first. She refused to be tested even when I pleaded with her. It was not until my aunt asked her, as a last request just before she died, that she finally had the testing done.

Sharon Larsen

It took me two years from being told I have the BRCA2 mutation to get it all done, but I felt I was ready. I'm glad. I look at it this way: I'm lucky to have been given this valuable information and have the chance to have this surgery and hopefully stop it from developing. Unfortunately, my Aunty didn't get this chance. With this I say, thank you, Aunty Daphne. I love you...RIP

Carrie Gaspar Katai

It wasn't until I started getting to the age that my mom was first diagnosed with breast cancer at twenty-nine that I really began thinking seriously about my BRCA gene.

Stephanie Bangel

At the age of twenty-seven, I asked my doctor his thoughts about BRCA testing. His advice was not to be tested, because if I did indeed test positive, I would live my life just waiting for the cancer to take me over. That was stupid. Now, I tell everyone I know that has a family history of cancer that they should talk to their doctor about BRCA testing. I have a donation box on the counter at my candy store for the Revlon Run/Walk For Women[73]. It's there all year 'round and is the catalyst to many conversations about the cause.

Susan Lugibihl-Swenson

I, at age fifty-three, just had a preventative mastectomy in which they did find DCIS. I also had my ovaries and fallopian tubes removed.

The BRCA2 mutation runs in my family. We learned of it this year. I encouraged my then twenty-five-year-old daughter to have genetic counseling at the Mayo Clinic. My daughter was told she has the BRCA2 genetic mutation. She had preventative mastectomy within a month. It took her very little time to decide this was the right thing to do, given she saw her aunt, my sister, live through breast cancer.

Teri
I'm Anti-Cancer

"I am not pro-surgery. I'm anti-cancer."

Amy S.

Nothing against doctors, but the ones I've worked with have a hard time acknowledging they can make mistakes and that horses really can be zebras sometimes.

Krystin Tate

We couldn't choose to have this mutation or not, but we are choosing what we do with it and a lot of amazing things are happening in the process.

Raechel Maki

Well, there was no known BRCA mutation in my family prior to me. The only incidence of breast or ovarian cancer in our family was my mother who was diagnosed stage IIIC ovarian cancer at the age of forty-seven and died at fifty-one. She was never BRCA tested, even after her diagnosis. I had hyst/BSO about a year after finding out my status, and just one month ago had my NSBPM. And now, I am relieved.

Suhir Jibreen

I feel very positive about the whole thing now, and although it changes my future somewhat, I strongly feel I have been put in a great position, enabling me to take control and also actually giving me a choice, which is a far cry from what many were given.

Sharon Larsen

I finally went through with my hysterectomy. I'm still recovering, and well, I might add. I feel a weight has been lifted. I'm due to go back to my gyn next week for a checkup. I'll be back to work in two weeks.

Stephanie Bangel

The advice I would give someone is simple: Take care of yourself and don't wait to find out about something that could have been prevented earlier. Don't miss an opportunity.

Lulu Luke

The biggest shock for the family was finding out that my mum didn't have the gene mutation and that it came from my dad instead.

Note from Teri About Lulu's Comments: *Once again busting open the fallacy that men don't have to concern themselves with this topic!*

Lulu Luke

My genetic nurse retired, so I applied for her job. I now work as a breast care nurse in the breast cancer family history clinic and the national screening program.

Sue Kuck-Junkert

Two years after my BRCA positive results, I did have a total hysterectomy. I was postmenopausal, in very good health, my children were gainfully employed and on their own. I was not ready to for the PBM. Then, I was diagnosed with breast cancer of the left breast at age fifty-three.

Pat Martin

My mother was diagnosed with breast cancer at the age of thirty-six. This was in the seventies. Four years later, she developed a new cancer in her ovaries. The doctors at that time were amazed and wrote her up in a medical journal because of this.

She died at the age of forty-four. That was twenty-seven years ago.

Rosie G.

Dear Doctor, approximately five years into my treatment, I asked you if my being an Ashkenazi Jew could have anything to do with my ovarian cancer. The look on your face was priceless! As part of the intake process, why wasn't I asked about family history or background?

Karen Malkin-Lazarovitz

I can only imagine how hard it is for a parent to know their children have this. I have a son and a daughter, and I hope beyond hope that they are negative. That might not be the case. I only hope they know I did what I did not only for me but also for them.

Pat Martin

A piece of my heart breaks a bit for all of the survivors and Previvors I read about. What a battle we all are fighting! I see things in life a lot clearer. I have a new appreciation for the small stuff. And believe me, I give thanks each day for another day on this earth.

Sara Bartosiewicz-Hamilton

In a way, knowing I'm BRCA2 positive was almost a relief. Our entire lives, we watched so many of our family members fight cancer...some winning, others not.

Amy Shainman

My view is that I simply removed the parts of me that were causing more harm than good.

Sara Bartosiewicz-Hamilton

To now have something to point to and feel as though I can take more control by changing my lifestyle, being proactive in screening, I feel like maybe I can have some say rather than just waiting around, hoping cancer doesn't find me. Don't get me wrong; I'm still terrified to get cancer, but to know why, it gave me some odd form of clarity and/or comfort.

Teri's Blog

BRCA really took over my life, but mostly in a good way. Being BRCA positive has helped me grow as a person, and I found this inner philanthropist I never knew was there. I built a name for myself within the BRCA community because I care. And I care passionately.

Kathleen Cordero

I want my doctors to stay current. It's great that they know what my odds for each of the cancers are. But tell me what's happening with the latest research. Many of us keep up with the research, and as for me, I'd like to discuss that latest research with my doctor. It might not help us right now, but it could very well help our daughters and our friends.

Lisa Grocott

I also have been telling my doctors about the *Prepare for Surgery, Heal Faster*[74] book and have been pleasantly surprised at how open some are for recognizing the validity of offering patients this kind of support, especially when they can see patients who have felt cheated by their bodies and need a way to turn around their negative thoughts into positive future images of themselves once they have healed.

Kay Edwards

I had my ten-hour surgery, bilateral mastectomies with *lat-dorsi* reconstruction. When the tissue went away to be checked, I got the news that I was in the right place at the right time, because they found a small tumor in each side, small enough to not need any further treatment, thankfully.

Raechel Maki

I can be an inspiration for others to be proactive about their own health and cancer predisposition by encouraging genetic testing and making myself available to those who are thinking about going through all of this and have questions.

Teri

My thoughts to doctors from the perspective of a BRCA mutant: This may be routine to you, but to your patient, it's very likely all new, confusing and frightening. Please treat them with compassion and respect. Explain what is happening in terms they can understand. Yes, we know you're super smart, but talk to us in language we can follow. I'm not saying to "dumb it down," but don't use big words to make yourself sound smarter; big words we don't understand just confuse us further!

Be honest. If you don't know much about the subject, admit it! Either learn what you can, or recommend us to someone who does know about it. These are our lives we are talking about.

We know you have resources we don't. Please have your administrative staff help us figure out the insurance aspect of prophylactic surgeries. We have enough on our minds wondering if we're going to get cancer and die before we have to cut our breasts off and our ovaries out! Your billing department knows all about how to code procedures so insurance companies will pay. Please help us with this, and let us know you're doing so!

Please, stay up to date on the latest information! There are still doctors out there who are telling women that estrogen replacement is harmful to them and shouldn't be used at any cost! There are still doctors telling women that the BRCA mutation cannot be passed on paternally! There are still doctors who insist men can't get breast cancer. This is misinformation! There are women needlessly suffering because their doctor isn't up to date on current studies.

Margaret Tueller-Proffitt

The good news is that at least I know about it. My grandmother died from breast cancer, my mother will beat it and, God willing, I'll never have to face it, because I know and I will be prepared.

Rebecca Amy Stenning-White

Being tested has given me some peace of mind and I feel in control of my future.

The Gift

Inspired by Vicki Little (New Zealand)

I am not a victim, I don't need your sympathy
I am my own woman, please give me room to breathe
Although this thing inside of me, has taken part of me
This is not who I am, nor who I want to be
I am who I was before, and who I will always be
The scars I bear are mine alone
They cannot be shared, nor be undone
The price I paid, the price for life
A gift I gave, a sacrifice
A nervous strength that pushed me through
Awaits the approving silence, if they only knew
The path I chose, I walk alone
The ones I love, all stand in toe
The light ahead, it seems so far
The path behind is just as far.
I know one day I will find some peace
The pain, the hurt, will be released
The scars will fade, thoughts forgotten
That path ahead will be wide open
I chose to live, without a shadow to hang over me
A life to share with my friends and family
And now here starts a new chapter in the life of me
With Strength and youth, and vitality
I thank you all from the very heart of me

~~ Paul Nelson

Citations & Endnotes

[1] National Institute of Health (NIH) http://www.nih.gov/

[2] American Society of Clinical Oncology (ASCO), http://www.asco.org/

[3] Teri's Blip in the Universe, blog by Teri Smieja, retrieved 09/30/2013, http://myblip.wordpress.com/

[4] http://www.cancer.gov/cancertopics/factsheet/Risk/BRCA#r5

[5] http://www.cancer.gov/cancertopics/factsheet/Risk/BRCA#r5

[6] http://www.facebook.com/groups/brcasisterhood/, BRCA Sisterhood Facebook Group

[7] http://www.facingourrisk.org/, Facing Our Risk Empowered, FORCE

[8] https://www.facebook.com/ChaseCommunityGiving Chase Community Giving Campaign

[9] http://losingtheboobs.blogspot.com/2010/04/21-baukje-macinnishommersen-nee-klaver.html?zx=b6eaa34665b3a6a3

[10] https://www.stephencovey.com/, Dr. Stephen Covey

[11] Lennox Hill Hospital, http://www.lenoxhillhospital.org/

[12] New York Eye and Ear Infirmary, https://www.nyee.edu/

[13] The New York Center for the Advancement of Breast Reconstruction http://www.nyee.edu/ny-center-for-the-advancement-of-breast-reconstruction.html

[14] Learnabouthboc.com, Lecture available in archives

[15] American Society of Clinical Oncology, http://www.asco.org/, retrieved 10/04/2013

[16] Published guidelines are available from the Association of Community Cancer Centers (ACCC), American Congress of Obstetrics and Gynecologists (ACOG), American Medical Association (AMA, American Society of Breast Surgeons (ASBC), American Society of Clinical Oncology (ASCO), The National Comprehensive Cancer Network (NCCN), The Society of Surgical Oncology (SSO), Society of Gynecologic Oncologists (SGO), and the U.S. Preventive Services Task Force (USSTF).

[17] http://www.cancer.org/cancer/breastcancer/detailedguide/breast-cancer-risk-factors

[18] http://www.aetna.com/

[19] Retrieved 10/01/2013, https://www.brocadestudy.com/?mm_campaign=aab5df3bf54aae6be77fe0f 00cc61350&gclid=CMLzxabu_bkCFUVk7AodiX0AqA

[20] Siegel R., Naishadham D., Jemal A. Cancer Statistics, 2012. *CA Cancer J Clin.* 2012;62:10-29.

[21] http://www.cancer.gov/dictionary?cdrid=45978, Retrieved 09/28/2013

[22] Retrieved, 10/1/2013, http://www.cancer.org/cancer/breastcancer/detailedguide/breast-cancer-risk-factors

[23] Retrieved 09/30/2013, http://www.nice.org.uk/nicemedia/live/13464/57792/57792.pdf, April 2011, Developed for NICE by the National Collaborating Centre for Cancer

[24] Risk Assessment Form for Hereditary Cancers, http://www.myriad.com/lib/risk-assessment/medonc-ra.pdf

[25] http://www.nlm.nih.gov/medlineplus/druginfo/meds/a682414.html

[26] http://www.nlm.nih.gov/medlineplus/druginfo/meds/a698007.html

[27] http://www.avastin.com/patient

[28] http://www.nhlbi.nih.gov/whi/

[29] http://www.climara-us.com/index.html

[30] http://www.cmdrc.com/middle-to-transition-years/menopause

[31] Koushik et al. Characteristics of menstruation and pregnancy and the risk of lung cancer in women. International Journal of Cancer, 2009 DOI: 10.1002/ijc.24560

[32] http://www.premarin.com/index

[33] Breast Reconstruction Options, Cancer.org, http://www.cancer.org/cancer/breastcancer/moreinformation/breastreconstructionaftermastectomy/breast-reconstruction-after-mastectomy-toc

[34] http://www.breastcenter.com/ Center for Restorative Breast Surgery in New Orleans

[35] https://www.facebook.com/pages/Patient-Empowerment-Program-NYBRA-at-Aesthetic-Plastic-Surgery-PC/168444969860721

[36] Breastreconstruction.org

[37] http://www.cancer.gov/cancertopics/factsheet/Sites-Types/paget-breast

[38] http://www.nhs.uk, National Health Service, United Kingdom

[39] http://www.amazon.com/Breast-Reconstruction-Guidebook-Second-Edition/dp/0966979974

[40] http://www.lifecell.com/health-care-professionals/lifecell-products/allodermr-regenerative-tissue-matrix/applications-and-procedures/breast-reconstruction/

[41] Double Fantasy (1980), John Lennon

[42] Hereditary breast cancer in Jews. Rubinstein WS. Fam Cancer. 2004;3(3-4):249-57. Review. PMID: 15516849 [PubMed - indexed for MEDLINE]

[43] "Approximately 2,200 men per year get breast cancer." Cancer.org, http://www.cancer.org/cancer/breastcancerinmen/detailedguide/breast-

cancer-in-men-key-statistics, retrieved 09/30/2013
[44] http://www.healthit.gov/buzz-blog/electronic-health-and-medical-records/emr-vs-ehr-difference/
[45] http://www.northshorelij.com/hospitals/location/division-plastic-reconstructive-surgery
[46] http://www.northshorelij.com/hospitals/location/lij-medical-center
[47] http://www.drphil.com/
[48] http://www.comcast.com/corporate/shop/products/local/pennsylvania/pa/philadelphia.html
[49] MacGuffin Films http://www.macguffin.com/
[50] http://www.uabmedicine.org/conditions-and-services/interventional-radiology-mediport-placement Information about Mediports and other medical port placement procedures.
[51] Sloan Kettering, http://www.mskcc.org/
[52] http://www.ucsf.edu/ University of California, San Francisco
[53] http://breastcenter.ucla.edu/body.cfm?id=33 UCLS High-Risk Program for women.
[54] http://www.drorringer.com/
[55] http://www.911memorial.org/ September 11, 2001, Terrorist attacks collapse United State's and results in collapse of the World Trade Center towers and the pentagon.
[56] http://shobgyn.com/home/splash.php
[57] http://piwhdenver.com/our_providers
[58] http://www.plannedparenthood.org/ Planned Parenthood
[59] http://www.ucdenver.edu/pages/ucdwelcomepage.aspx
[60] http://www.upstate.edu/com/about/campuses/bing/

[61] http://www.ethicon.com/ Ethicon Endo-surgery
[62] American Cancer Society. Cancer Facts & Figures 2011. Atlanta: American Cancer Society, Inc. retrieved from,
http://www.breastcancerdeadline2020.org/breast-cancer-information/specific-issues-in-breast-cancer/dcis/ 09/30/2013
[63] "Prevalence of BRCA1 and BRCA2 Mutations in Women Diagnosed With Ductal Carcinoma In Situ", Elizabeth B. Claus, MD, PhD; Stacey Petruzella, MS, MPH; Ellen Matloff, MS; Darryl Carter, MD, JAMA. 2005;293(8):964-969. doi:10.1001/jama.293.8.964
[64] http://www.amh.org/AHPhysicians/Practices/apwhg/#.UIJGsxARXyU
[65] http://www.nccn.org/index.asp, Guidelines:
http://www.nccn.org/professionals/physician_gls/f_guidelines.as
[66] http://www.facingourrisk.org/FORCE_community/previvors.php, Previvorship and the term Previvor, coined and trademarked by FORCE.
[67] H.Res. 1522 (111th): Expressing support for designation of the last week of

September as National Hereditary Breast and Ovarian Cancer
www.govtrack.us/congress/bills/111/hres1522/text/ih
[68] http://www.amazon.com/Confronting-Hereditary-Breast-Ovarian-Cancer/dp/1421404087
[69] FORCE annual conference:
http://www.facingourrisk.org/events/annual_conference/index.php
[70] http://www.penncancer.org/basser/
[71] To contact a qualified genetics expert, visit the FORCE website on genetic counseling or speak with a board-certified genetic counselor at FORCE's "Ask-A-Counselor" toll-free helpline (866-288-7475, ext. 704).,
http://www.facingourrisk.org/
[72] Five Stages of Grieving, Axelrod, Julie, retrieved 9/30/2013,
http://psychcentral.com/lib/the-5-stages-of-loss-and-grief/000617
[73]Revlon Run/Walk for Woman website and donation information.
http://do.eifoundation.org/site/PageNavigator/2013_runwalk_splash.html
[74] Prepare for Surgery, Heal Faster, by Peggy Huddleston, a book and workshop designed to help people heal better and faster, as a whole, after surgical procedures. http://www.healfaster.com/

71939459R00174

Made in the USA
Columbia, SC
07 June 2017